THE SUCC

"After reading The on my 100 day pr\ *already "richer" - but this book, The Success...*
Gets Rich! has inspired me further to be more in control of finances, to wish for "more than enough" and get it, and has taught me that there is more to just making money. I learned a lot about some of the groundwork of taking care of my future and my children's future!" ~Nanette Labastida, Realtor, Austin, TX

"This book isn't just a collection of stories and cliché examples, this book is packed full of tactical steps to finding your dreams and following them. Any single mom who is struggling to figure out what to do next needs to read this book. There is tactical advice paired up with inspirational stories from real single moms who have been there and done that. Honoree gives hope to every single mom who just can't quite figure out where to go from here." ~Cassie Boorn, Blogger & Social Media Specialist, Illinois

"The Successful Single Mom Gets Rich! was written to inspire and guide single moms (and married ones too) to becoming successful and rich! Even as a married mother this book is a must read. From juggling it all without dropping a ball, to living the life you became a Mom to have, this book will show you the way to a truly prosperous life." ~Joan C. Richardson, JCR Enterprises, LLC, Dallas, Texas

About <u>The Successful Single Mom</u>

"I've been able to change my life and my future with Honorée's help and the tools from this book!" ~Christine Plaisted, Participant in The Successful Single Mom Group

"This book is for all single mothers who want to get their mojo back, feel empowered, get focused and be in control of their own destiny." ~Julie A. Booth, Participant in The Successful Single Mom Group

"Honorée's Successful Single Mom Transformation Program helped me get my life back on track. Finally a guide for single moms everywhere!" ~Melinda Payne, Participant in The Successful Single Mom Group

"This book has the potential to lift you from the depths of despair to the heights of self-empowered living. It is a must-read for every single mom." ~Alisa McAffee, Participant in The Successful Single Mom Group

"<u>The Successful Single Mom</u> has a lot to offer the newly-divorced mother in regard to personal and professional goal-setting after divorce. The author is honest about the feelings of fear and rejection that accompany the end of a marriage and the emotional paralysis that can result. That said, the book moves quickly from acknowledging those feelings, getting whatever help is necessary from professionals, clergy or friends and planning a future for you and your children. This book will be particularly

THE SUCCESSFUL SINGLE MOM GETS RICH!

TAKE CONTROL OF YOUR FINANCES AND YOUR FUTURE

HONORÉE CORDER

Published by Honorée Enterprises Publishing, LLC.

Copyright 2011-2013 ©Honorée Enterprises
Publishing, LLC & Honorée Corder

ISBN 978-0991669608

Discover other titles by Honorée Corder at http://www.
coachhonoree.com, Amazon.com, BarnesandNoble.com,
Smashwords.com and on iBooks.

helpful to women who want to start their own business. The author has much to offer in this area as she ran her own business before her divorce and shares a number of her keys to building and maintaining a successful business. In addition, she has developed a 100-Day Plan, complete with worksheets, to encourage women to begin setting goals for themselves. This plan, however, is not for everyone as each woman must find her own way and the pace that works for her. A large part of the divorce experience is learning about yourself and developing your own style for creating a life for you and your family. Whatever choices you eventually make, this book will get you thinking and moving!" ~Jeanne L. Ward, Author: You're It! Successful Single Mothering After Divorce (Amazon Review)

"This is the best book for anyone who needs some help finding direction in their life. The author has a great sense of humor and is able to connect with the reader. The tools and techniques are not overwhelming or intimidating and are easy to put into practice. I highly recommend this book to anyone starting out on a new adventure in life." ~K. Russell, Rochester, NY (Amazon Review)

"Honorée's latest book is a must read for any woman looking for success. This book gives inspiration, direction, and practical advice on how to get your life back on track while still maintaining warmth and humor throughout. Honorée's coaching style is direct and right on target – she hones in on what needs to be done and how to do it, while still recognizing the challenges life throws your way. I find myself reading and re-reading it. I'd recommend this

to anyone who's ready to take charge, make changes, and actually enjoy themselves in the process!" ~Nicole Dupre, Rubber Duckie Creations (Amazon Review)

"I'm not even recently divorced, but 7 years later I still feel like I'm trying to figure out my life and my parenting. Everyone needs a cheerleader to keep you motivated and to boost your self-esteem. This is like a cheerleader in book form! I carry it in my purse to remind me. This book is so perfect because it's a quick and easy read (single parents don't have time to read!) and it has steps that are do-able and yet life-altering. Just what I needed." ~Nanette Scalzo, Austin, TX (Amazon Review)

Check out all the titles in The Successful Single Mom book series:

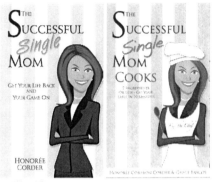

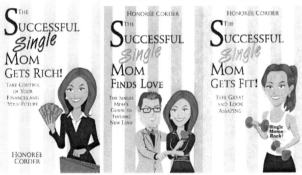

Coming soon:

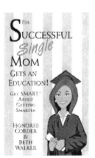

DEDICATION

Dedicated to you – the single mom. I wrote this book for you so you could thrive instead of struggle, and begin right now to be in control of your financial present and future. Cheers to you, your children and your future!

The best is yet to come.

TABLE OF CONTENTS

Dear Reader,

Single moms can be rich! Rich has many meanings; it's not just about the money. To me, being rich means there is more than enough to buy the basics (food, clothing and shelter), save, invest, vacation, have desired extras, live happily, and look forward to the future.

It is important to say this (again, if you've read The Successful Single Mom), right now at the very beginning: you don't become a "rich successful single mom" – you already are one! You are rich because you're alive, you have a wonderful child or children, and you can still smile (sometimes through the tears). What I really want for you is to be right here, right now, enjoying the journey, feeling alive and creating what you want.

The single moms I know want to provide a solid, stress-free life for themselves and their children. This book will provide the basic knowledge you need, both mental and financial, to do just that.

What I won't cover are complex financial and legal concepts. You need a strong team that includes a seasoned financial advisor, and insurance, banking and tax professionals. If you run, or plan to run your own business, you'll need a business attorney. Once you have accumulated some wealth, you'll need an estate planning attorney and perhaps some others. Don't worry about that yet; just start right where you are and bloom from there.

I've struggled and I've thrived. Thriving is easier, keeps stress levels down and makes being a fun, happy mom easier. This book will help you to get where you want to go faster, and I hope you enjoy it.

To your best success,

Honorée Corder
Author, Speaker, Coach, Mom

MEET THE MOMS

I had the pleasure of interviewing some of the most amazing women on the planet, who also happen to be successful single moms. These ladies achieved their greatest success after becoming single moms, some of them after experiencing and enduring tragedies, unspeakable challenges, and average every day disappointments. You will find yourself in some or all of them, and their stories will be covered in depth throughout the book.

Aljolynn Sperber – mom to Aidan (Irish for "little fire ball"), age 3. Aljolynn has been a single mom almost from the moment she discovered she was pregnant. After reaching her first goal of supporting her son without outside help, she joined forces with a girlfriend to start her own PR company. Now she has a solid income, savings, and is able to provide what she calls "the extras" for her son. You can find her online through her website: http://www.MarketingMavenPR.com, and on twitter: @MarketingMaven2.

Christine Plaisted – mom to Jack, age 16, and Roger, age 18. Christine owns her business, Mercury Permit Services in Las Vegas. Christine is now the ultimate optimist and hopes the single moms reading this book will find the courage to step out on their own, as she did, and know that they can do whatever they set their minds to. Follow her on twitter: @wyndsong, and get more info on her business http://www.mercurypermits.com.

Julie Booth – mom to Hannah, age 7. Julie has been able to successfully break away from her old CPA partnership during the 100 day program spelled out in The Successful Single Mom book, is now happily contracting with a respectable CPA firm, and has accumulated an excellent book of clients. This has allowed Julie to free up her schedule and spend the much-needed time with Hannah, as well as maintain a wonderful, secure life for them both. You can connect with Julie on LinkedIn: http://linkd.in/sMQOMc.

Tracy Shields – mom to two sons. Tracy's inspirational story includes the plan she put in place to leave her marriage, including getting her degree and ultimately run a large, successful company.

Nancy Butler – mom to 2 grown children, Nancy's daughters were 8 and 15 at the time of her divorce. Now a retired multi-millionaire who travels the world and does inspirational talks, Nancy started over without even a personal identity! With hard work and determination, she not only learned about the world of saving and investing, she eventually owned the company! Find her online at her website: http:www.aboveallelse.org, on twitter: @NJButler1, on facebook: http://tinyurl.com/78zj3ct, and on LinkedIn: http://tinyurl.com/7944rsh.

Kristen Brown – mom to Brooke, age 5, she's the Widow Mom Turned Queen of Stress Relief and Bestselling Author! Just thirty years old when her young husband died suddenly, Kristen turned tragedy into triumph as she made powerful personal decisions that changed the course of her life, and the lives of many others, for the better. Visit her website: http://www.HappyHourEffect.com, Read her bestseller: The Best Worst Thing, listen to her show: The

Happy Hour Effect with Kristen Brown, follow her on twitter @HappyHourEffect, and read her blog: http://site.happyhoureffect.com/blog/.

Julie Pech – mom to a 14-year-old and 16-year-old. She's The Chocolate Therapist and she writes, speaks and lectures all around the world on the benefits of chocolate. Making a giant leap of faith into single motherhood and self-employment, Julie is a excellent example of what's possible for all single moms! Follow her on twitter: @chocolateluvr, find her on facebook: http://on.fb.me/t1NBxc, connect with her on LinkedIn: http://linkd.in/tN2tuK.

Nanette Labastida -- mom to Claudia 13, Gabriel 9. A single mom for seven years, she's also a one-year breast cancer survivor! Buy a house in Austin, Texas: http://rocknrealty.net/, Read her blog: http://www.glittereveryday.blogspot.com, find her on facebook: http://www.facebook.com/eastaustinhomes, and follow her on twitter @Rocknrealty.

Cassie Boorn – mom to Aiden, age 5, has an incredible story of teen pregnancy to college education and enviable employment. You can find out more about Cassie on her blog: http://www.cassieboorn.com, and follow her on twitter: @cassieboorn.

PROLOGUE

How will I ever support my little one? That thought is always in the back of your mind as a single mom. You don't just have a lack of an extra set of hands, you also lack that extra set of hand's paycheck.

It's challenging enough with two parents to pay the bills, at times, unless you're in a very elite class of earners. If you have an advanced degree and a great job, you stand a great chance of earning a sufficient, or even terrific, living.

Sadly, that isn't the life of most single moms. It certainly wasn't my case! I had barely graduated high school, not because I wasn't smart and capable, but because I had endured an abusive father and an indifferent mother. I felt like I was in a fight for my life (because I was), so my grades reflected what was happening at home. Even eventually going to college (especially since my parents weren't exactly going to pay for it) was the last thing on my mind.

My parents did do one thing right, however, they encouraged entrepreneurship. Being from the Midwest, where hard work is the model, I learned hard work is the way to go. My father always said, "If you're working for someone, you're working for the Pharaoh, someone is going to get rich and it's not going to be you. Do yourself a favor and work for yourself."

Well, without a college degree, that was pretty much my only option anyway. That was my belief, and our beliefs become reality, right? I believed without an advanced education, there was only so far I could go in the corporate world and therefore in life. I was both right and wrong.

At the age of 22, I started my own networking marketing business. It took a few years, and many tears, to find my way. But when I did, it was amazing! I made a large income, discovered how to run a successful business and through that process, discovered some of life secrets (which I'm now delighted to share with you).

You see success is based on a few very fundamentals. Jim Rohn, the father of the personal development movement, says there are 6, 7, 8, maybe 10 at most. You don't have to know a lot of complex, complicated, hard-to-understand principles, just a few. When you know them, and execute them on a regular basis, you will be successful.

It's time for you to raise the bar about what you expect for yourself.

This book includes the Single Mom Prosperity Principles. The principles I believe, when executed, will all but ensure you'll be as financially sound as you want to be.

Are you ready? Read on!

THE SUCCESSFUL SINGLE MOM
PROSPERITY PRINCIPLES

1. Where are you now?

2. Anything is possible!

3. Ask for Expert Help & Expand Your Knowledge

4. Create Your Plan

5. Get busy!

6. Stay Focused

7. See it, Do it, Show it. Educate your kids about money, too!

8. Enjoy the process.

CHAPTER ONE

ANYTHING IS POSSIBLE

"A woman is like a tea bag: you cannot tell how strong she is until you put her in hot water."
~Eleanor Roosevelt

According to the 2010 Census, there are 9.9 million single mothers in the U.S. These ladies face challenges many other moms and dads don't. Between managing work and home, financial commitments and extracurricular activities, a single mom's work - alone - is never done.

In addition, most single moms experience a dramatic decrease in their standard of living after a divorce. Statistics show that women experience a 27 percent decrease in their standard of living, while the men have a 10 percent standard of living increase the first year after divorce. I'm not one to dwell on statistics, but I think it's helpful to have a clear picture.

The good news: that doesn't have to be your story. It might be for a time or even right now, depending upon your circumstances. Whether you've been divorced for a minute or even many years, if you're still struggling it is understandable that you would still be having a hard time. It's even expected! Single moms haven't had a stigma for the past fifty years for nothing!

However, it doesn't have to be or stay your reality. I promise.

One of the reasons I wrote this book is because I believe that regardless of where you start out, anything is possible for you. I want you to start to believe it, and eventually to know it.

I want you to have the tools, strategies and resources to create whatever you want to create. It is possible to achieve your goals, regardless of whether your goals are to be able to support your children with enough money to go to the movies once a month, or to become a millionaire and retire in a few years. In this book, you'll read about moms who have done both – and everything in between.

I've experienced a complete financial transformation since my divorce without the benefit of family support, a college education or even a basic accounting class. I didn't know what I didn't know, so I made some interesting mistakes and had long, unnecessary delays. Yet I've triumphed in spite of my challenges and very simply, if I can do it, so can you. I want to shorten your journey to financial success and help you avoid some delays and landmines along the way.

Don't get me wrong: It's not only about the money. A rich life is full of everything you need, including money. But this book is specifically about getting rich, securing your financial future so you can act from a place of power. Not having enough, almost having enough, having just enough, having more than enough, and having more than enough so you can share what's left over. All of those situations feel differently, and having been in all of those places, I know for a fact decisions are made differently when you're in each of those positions.

I've heard, "I don't need millions of dollars ..." Great, and that's true, you don't. But there's no shame in wanting millions of dollars. There's no shame in wanting to have just enough to support your kids and be able to have the occasional treat. If you're reading this book, I can assume you want to make a positive leap in your financial circumstances, and I'm here to help you get it.

Just know that I'm not "all about the money," but what I know for sure is that having an abundance of it is helpful in many ways. It's psychologically reassuring to have a reserve, and eventually, a war chest. It allows you to make your most important life choices from the best possible place.

What does that mean, being able to make choices from a positive place? Well, I've been in more than a few conversations with ladies – and not just single moms – who were in, or who had stayed in, relationships because they knew they would have a hard time without "his income." They put up with crap, settled for less than they deserved, and in many cases felt helpless because they didn't have enough or more than enough to leave, to start over, to do what their heart desired.

If you're ready, you can now begin to see what you've been doing, even been settling for, and make some steps in the direction you'd really like to go.

So what. Now what?

Your past and your present don't necessarily predict your future, but they do shape it. We certainly make decisions based upon our points of reference. In fact, many of our actions are automatic because of them! This means that what we saw our parents do and believe around wealth and money, we tend to do ourselves. If our parents believed there was always plenty to go around, we will tend to believe that, too. If they were scared or worried about money, we will tend to do that, too.

My mother was always concerned and worried about money, and my father was always obsessed with making money. My mother would use grocery money for other things, like clothes or extras. My father was envious and jealous of people who had money, and when he had money, he bought lots for himself but almost nothing for his family.

What I learned from them was, frankly, a scarcity mentality. Once I realized I was modeling what I learned, I got to step back and evaluate whether being worried about money all the time was effective or ineffective for me. You get to do the same!

Based on my upbringing, it was no surprise that I married into a less-than-abundant situation. I married a divorced military man with three children, tons of debt and a large child support payment. Because of that, we struggled for years. I learned to do without, settle, and live in a constant state of stress. Several things blasted me out of this lack and limitation, and I've used those tools and strategies throughout the years to continually expand my beliefs and reality. (Don't worry; my personal strategies are covered in this book!)

Thankfully, I was able to get myself to a state of abundance by being open to the possibilities and finding out what worked for me through trial and error. Then I remarried, and my current husband Byron has taught me a lot about thinking even bigger and more abundantly.

For example, I used to shop on a "need to buy" basis. If I "needed" M&Ms, I would buy a single serving pack. If I send my husband to buy M&Ms (or anything else for that matter), he buys the two-pound bag! Then he'll say, "Well, you'll eat them eventually won't you?"

He learned this abundant thinking from his mom. Right after we were married, I asked her to pick me up a lint roller at the grocery store. She came back with twelve!

My thinking was, "I don't need twelve, I need one." But wouldn't you know, since I've had them, I've used them! Watching my husband and his mom caused me to stop and think about why I never bought more than I needed, from having one pair of basic black heels to almost running out of toilet paper all the time because I didn't buy more than one pack at a time.

Because of these shifts, when I shop now, I always buy more than enough. The interesting thing is that there's always enough money to support me buying what I need. What I've learned, modeled and observed is all connected. I know that now, but I sure didn't know that before.

I have had the opportunity to expand my thinking, and in doing so, I've noticed it's positively affected other areas of my life, too.

Not "Right or Wrong" … "Effective or "Ineffective"

As a coach, I don't live in a world of "right" or "wrong." I think it's much better to decide if something is "effective" or "ineffective."

Is what you're doing and believing about and around money, wealth, and abundance effective or ineffective for you? Said another way, do you have enough? Do you have more than enough? Are you able to pay the bills with plenty left over? If not, would you like to experience what that it is like to have more than enough?

If so, you must first surrender the past to the past, analyze your beliefs, decide what you want, and get ready for an amazing future.

Didn't I just make the process sound so easy? In some

ways, it really is! If you're ready, let's get started.

THE PAST

If you don't have one yet, grab a journal or download a notebook app onto your iPad (I use NotesPlus and Penultimate).

- What did I see my parents doing regarding money?

- What did my parents believe about money?

- Is what was modeled for me what I want to recreate in my life?

- Is what I'm modeling for my kids what I want them to create in their lives?

Now, if you're like me, the answer to the last two questions is a resounding no. I didn't, and don't, want a life of continuous struggle, stress and strain. That's what was modeled for me and I didn't realize how what is modeled is what can happen, but doesn't have to happen.

I want a life of ease and abundance. Maybe you do, too?

Again, if you're like me, that may require a shift in beliefs and actions to create the desired results. If your parents modeled great things, perhaps it's time you live into that for yourself, if you're not doing that now.

Let me say that this process is about you and what you want. There's no right or wrong about that, it just is what it is – and it's either effective or ineffective. You can want what you want and whatever you want is just fine! Know that, and then let's proceed.

THE PRESENT

Where are you now?

In order to get where you want to go, the first thing you need to do is to know exactly where you are today. As you begin to assemble your team, they will ask detailed questions so they know the best way to advise you. But let's not get ahead of ourselves!

For our purposes right now, the first order of business is to get clarity on where you are versus where you want to go.

More questions (grab that journal again):

- Do I know my net worth? If yes, what is it?

- Do I have debt, and if yes, how much?

- Do I have savings and investments? If yes, what are the current balances and values?

- What do I believe about money: there's always enough/just enough/never enough?

- Is what I believe effective or ineffective based upon what I'd truly like?

What did you discover? Perhaps that there's room for an 'upgrade?' I know, for me too. Just so you know, there's always room for an upgrade, if you want one.

Let's keep going!

THE FUTURE

Where do you want to go?

This is the fun part. If you're driving around in a 1972 Volkswagen Bug that breaks down every third turn of the road, worry not! You can, mentally, drive around in your shiny new 2012 Volkswagen Bug, Toyota Corolla, or Rolls Royce Phantom.

Whatever has come into your life has come into it mentally first. First you imagine going to the grocery store and buying bread, and then you do it. The same is true with your future, the future you want to create right now.

Before the questions, let me give you some important insight. The formula for success is:

Intention + Mechanism = Success.

Just out of curiosity, what percentage is intention and what percentage is mechanism? I bet the truth will surprise you: it's:

100% Intention + 0% Mechanism = 100% Success

Really? Yes, really.

So before you go any further, just know that when you're 100% committed to your intention, the mechanism isn't your concern. What and who you need will show up, cross your path, come to you.

In case this sounds too "woo woo" or "out there" for you, don't worry. I'm all about getting the mind right, but I also believe you've got to move your ass, too, in order for things to happen. So we'll get your mind right and we'll also make sure you're taking the right actions.

Single Mom Aljolynn Sperber's Story

Aljolynn's single mom story begins before her son was even born. The father insisted she give the baby up for adoption, or consider an abortion. After consulting a counselor, Aljolynn realized that she really wanted to have her baby. She gave up a good-paying job to move closer to her family. The move led to a year of struggle while she figured out her options. When being close to family didn't go as planned, she took another chance and moved again. This time, she was offered a freelance position by a PR firm in Los Angeles, where she worked her way into a solid, full-time position helping to run the office. She earns a comfortable living for herself and son.

"I'm at a point now in my career that I am able to travel maybe once a month and not have to worry about my son's childcare being taken care of, paying extra money to the babysitter to watch him, and making sure there's enough at home to take care of him. I have life insurance in case something happens because I travel so much," she says. "Before that I couldn't travel or take client meetings or bring him a nice little souvenir back from my trips. I'm going to be gone for his birthday this year so I'm scheduling to have balloons and cupcakes at his daycare to celebrate his special day. Now I can pay for the extras, have a cushion, and I am able to do the extra stuff that I need or want."

She has some encouraging words, "Single parents in general are super heroes, I am amazed by what we're all able to accomplish. The PR company I work for is owned by my friend of 15 years. She is my boss, and the company has boomed because we love what we do. This proves that it's possible for a business to grow and succeed through a slow-growing economy. This is a true lesson in calculated risk taking and success. This, too, is true for single moms. If there's ever a time to take a risk, it's when it involves your future."

Now, your questions:

- What do you want to make (in total income, including but not limited to: your job, spousal/child support, interest income, residual income, referral fees, unexpected gifts, etc.)?

- Where do you want to live?

- How do you want to live?

- Who do you want to live with you?

- Where do you want to travel, visit, have other homes, explore?

- What do you want to do? If you could be paid to do anything and make an abundant living doing it, what would it be?

- Are you doing any or all of the above right now?

- Could you be doing more? If yes, what?

Now, wasn't that fun? I had fun just writing the questions because my mind started going crazy with ideas, thoughts, and inspirations. I hope yours is doing the same!

Coach' note: Your mind will if you let it, just like what you want can happen if you let it!

You Need a Plan

We're not going to get crazy and create your plan right here in chapter one. What we're going to do first is get clear about why you need a plan.

I hear all the time: "I've got my goals in my head." Seriously? In your head? That's great, but if you want them to come to fruition, you can't just think it; you've got to ink it!

Your goals really must be in writing! By in writing I mean type them out or write them out, whatever works best for you.

Creating your plan, in writing, allows you to gain a clarity that doesn't come just by thinking about it. You get to include all of the facets and aspects, including action steps, thereby increasing the likelihood it will happen.

I'm sure you've heard this advice before. Write your goals down. If they're not written down, they're just dreams. The same is true with your plan.

Writing things down sets off a chain of events that will change your life. I am a firm believer of writing down goals and plans. A firm believer. It's my intention for you to really understand the true explosive power of writing down what you want and the plan that goes with it.

We are told that we should always write our goals down, but the reasons why we should are not thoroughly explored. I suspect that's why statistics show that only 2% of Americans actually write down their goals and plans.

If you understand why you should do something, you're more likely to actually do it, right?

For example, we are told to drink the equivalent of eight glasses of water a day. I know that number is in debate, but bear with me. If I told you all the reasons why you should be, such as: easy absorption of vitamins and minerals, improved energy, longer lifespan, increased mental and physical performance, removal of toxics in the body, a more youthful appearance, lower blood pressure, reduced headaches, and so forth, and I expanded on those reasons, you would probably get in the habit of drinking eight glasses of water a day. If those reasons were not given, you probably would not be inclined to do so.

By really understanding why writing things down is so

crucial and understanding the reasoning and logic behind why you must write them down, you will become more adept to picking up that activity until it becomes a skill.

The benefits to writing your goals down are threefold:

1. It forces you to define clearly what you want. In essence, it forces you to get clarity, to really think it through.

2. It frees up your mental real estate, allowing your thinking to ascend to the next level.

3. It incorporates all three learning modalities and stimulates your innate, inborn creativity.

To discuss the power of writing down what you truly want, let's discuss one of the goals that my daughter has, which is to make as much money as possible without a job.

Now, let's clearly define her goal in the form of a clear question so she can find clear answers.

"How can I make around $200 this weekend without getting a job?"

Notice how I clearly defined the goal in terms of the amount of money I want to make, the time span, and the circumstances. By clearly defining these elements, the answers will fit the question.

Here are the answers she came up with:

1. Collect cans and bottles and take them to a recycling bin to trade them for money.

2. Hold a garage sale and sell your shoes, clothing, books, toys, DVDs, and other "stuff" that I (read: my

parents) don't need anymore.

3.   Offer to sell my mom's books.

4.   Do odd jobs around the house, or help my mom with her businesses.

5.   Buy candy at Costco (a wholesale store) and prepare to sell them individually at school.

6.   Buy Gatorade and ice and sell it at the park to walkers and joggers.

By clearly defining the goal, we were able to come up with multiple solutions. By writing down each solution, she freed up more room in her mind and stimulated creativity to come up with solutions that she never would've thought of before.

While she was writing down goal and solutions, she was using all three modes of learning: visual, audio and kinesthetic. She was seeing what she was writing, she was hearing it in her head as she was writing, and she was actually using her body when writing them down. You'll most likely have the same, or similar, experience.

People learn things differently. Some may learn better by seeing, some by hearing, some by doing, but by incorporating all three when writing, you use all your learning capabilities and that in turn, along with clarity, frees up room in the mind and stimulates massive creativity.

I can tell you that the "buying candy and selling it at school from Costco" idea stimulated her creativity and led to the "buy Gatorade and ice and sell it at the park" idea.

To further demonstrate the power of writing, let's take that goal and develop it even further by writing it down in the form of a clear question and writing down answers to it.

How can she maximize profits when selling Gatorade to thirsty athletes at parks?

1. Do research to see which day has the greatest number of people (thus, highest potential number of customers) and which park has the thirstiest joggers.

2. Offer a discount to first time buyers.

3. Reward loyal customers with a frequent purchase card – buy 10 get the next 1 free.

4. See which flavors people like and buy only those.

5. Have enough change ready.

6. Say "thank you."

7. Decide the ideal number of Gatorade bottles to bring.

8. Decide where to sell first, maybe the soccer field, then basketball courts, then tennis courts.

9. Find which park is the best place to sell.

10. Maybe diversify your products by selling snacks too.

11. Maybe diversify with water (didn't even think about water, but the profit margin for water is huge. (You can buy 50 bottles for 6 dollars at Costco)

12. You could even offer combinations of water and Gatorade to maximize revenue and to turnover inventory quickly.

When you write things down, the ideas start to flow like a river on paper, and you'll find them to be good ones too!

Do you ever wonder why the people who achieve their goals and plans are the ones that write them down?

They achieve their goals and plans because they got the goal out of their head. The goal expanded into a plan of action. Then the action plan became reality!

When you write down what's in your head, you free up the mental real estate to think of ways to accomplish what you want, which frees up even more mental real estate. Writing things down ultimately stimulates your creativity and the result is a really good idea with a concrete plan of action that can easily be implemented.

Ever wonder why great authors write great books? It's not because they're great authors.

Great authors write great books because they simply write!

They write one scene. Then that scene is out of their head, and they can now think of ideas on how to continue the storyline. As they do so and write the scene down, their creativity starts awakening, and they get trapped in a beautiful cycle.

People who never write their goals down always have them stuck in their head and they have no "room" to think of ideas on how to act on them.

The following are some exercises you can do to start getting into the habit of writing things down.

1. Journaling.

Keep a journal of your life. Motivational Speaker Anthony Robbins said, "If your life is worth living, it's worth recording." So true. Nobody can write the story of your life better than you. Take time to remember the good memories of your life and do them justice. Don't leave them to the chance of the fragile mind. Write down every detail using your five senses and do so on a nightly basis. You will find that you'll uncover things about yourself you never realized before.

2. Question and Answers.

Writing out a simple clear question and answers to it is another powerful, yet simple approach to get into the habit of writing things down. In the case of my daughter's goal, writing her goal in the form of a question led to pretty good ideas. A high school kid could easily make a hundred bucks in profit on a weekend using the solution found above.

3. Mind Mapping.

I was first introduced to mind mapping when I read Tony Buzan's book on the subject. I was blown away. It was very helpful. Mind mapping is an extremely powerful tool in terms of learning, brainstorming, and stimulating creativity.

It starts by you writing down a question, goal, or idea on the center of a piece of paper and circling it. Then you can start branching off answers, other ideas, or tangents by drawing lines from that center circle, writing down the other things that come to mind and circling them. Then you can expand from that circle or from other circles. Soon you will have a spider web of interconnected ideas.

For more information on mind mapping, you can use our trusty friend Google!

4. Your Own Pep Talk.

I think this step can be a fun and powerful tool to demonstrate the power of writing things down and can also get you into the habit of writing.

Most people nowadays are experts in self-criticism. To counter that thought process, try writing down a pep talk to yourself that you can refer to every time you need a boost.

Think of all the positive qualities you possess. Write them down! You know what's going to happen? You free up room in your brain for more good qualities, which you write those down too. You start becoming creative and write down things you've never seen in yourself, causing the floodgates to start to open.

The result will be a masterpiece about yourself that you never knew existed.

Cherish your masterpiece about you, and be sure to add to it daily to become your own personal pep talk.

Writing is magic. It has the power to touch other people, to transform lives, to move people to take action, and to accomplish monumental dreams.

So what are you waiting for? Get into the habit of writing down. Start writing down your goals.

I will now leave you with an exercise you can do that will transform your life from this day forward.

Step 1:

Write down one clear goal you would like to accomplish this year that will make the biggest impact on your life.

Step 2:

Write that goal down in the form of a **clear** question.

Step 3:

Write a list of answers on how you can accomplish the one goal you've chosen.

By doing these simple steps, you'll find that you will be more motivated to take action in accomplishing your goals, because they're not stuck in your head.

Write It Down -> Gets it Out of Your Head -> Write More Down -> Stimulates Your Creativity -> Great Ideas and Action Plans Start to Formulate -> Implement Them -> Achieve Your Goals.

Your dreams start to manifest the second you write them down, so write them down now. You'll be glad you did.

Successful Single Mom Tracy Shields' Story

Tracy Shields, a single mom of two boys since 2004, has an attitude to inspire any single mom, "I never considered myself unfortunate. I always took the road of gratitude, so no matter how low down on the ground I was, I was grateful for my two boys, for the roof over my head, for being given the things I was given, I always looked at the things I had vs. what I didn't. I also stopped the constant negative thinking: the grass is always greener, or I've got to have a husband, keep up with the Jones's, my kids are going to suffer because they are in a broken home. Don't believe and wouldn't teach my children those things."

Enduring an abusive relationship, her husband left the first time when she had a 2½ year old and was eight months pregnant. She knew if she didn't keep her wits about her and act intentionally, her future, and her son's futures would be negatively affected. It was important to her to start to accumulate assets and get an education, two things she knew would ensure she would be able to take care of her boys. So, Tracy took back her husband, and together they bought a house. While working toward her college degree, she worked, took care of her boys and their home, all while enduring on-going physical and emotional abuse from her husband.

"I learned from my mother the difference between immediate gratification and deferred gratification. I knew if I left my marriage today it would immediately cause less suffering, but I wasn't prepared to do that. I knew if I created a plan, paid my dues and planted my seeds, I would be doing so as a much smarter woman," Tracy shared with me.

At the very same time as she was getting her degree, her father passed away and she inherited his company and with it, enough money to buy her way out of her marriage. She hasn't looked back since, and has created an amazing life for herself and her boys, on her own terms.

Today, she's about giving back and helping women in trouble. "Many women imagine their escape from their marriages as something abrupt or extreme, some of us really should take the time to sew the ground before we reap. Some of us really need to plan for years to make sure that we are comfortable enough and can financially be on our own. That is just as viable a plan as leaving right now. I could stay and be abused because I had a plan and a goal."

Her ex lives a block and a half down the road. He started paying child support a year ago. They are able to co-parent her boys. Her company is doing very well, and has worked in the marketing department since 2006, and also serves on the Board of Directors.

She's also found love and is in a committed relationship. "We are living together, very happily. He's just a very good family man."

CHAPTER TWO

FISCALLY FABULOUS

"Your goal should be out of reach but not out of sight."
~Anita DeFrantz

The first step toward getting rich is to make some important decisions. Before I dive into the "technical" decisions, it's critically important to "go visionary" or "go to the end." While what's already happened in your life may not be the best to look back on, the future you're visualizing needs to excite you, compel you to action, and most importantly, make you feel incredible!

If today were the end of your life and you were happily looking back at what you've done, created and accomplished financially, what would you see? How would you have provided for your children and yourself? Where did you live? Where did you travel? How did you create magic moments for yourself and your family?

It's fun to create a series of movies in your mind about what you'll be looking back at someday, and going first to the end will help you to make decisions to go in that direction.

Of course there's a good chance that you will find love again, if that's something you want. At that time, you'll have the opportunity to make different choices and decisions. When love happens for you, because you've made solid, in advance decisions from your best place of personal power, you'll get to make new decisions from that same place.

The End

Carve out an hour, pull out your trusty journal and write down the script of your life as if it has already happened. You can include all aspects of your life, including another love and more children, how much money you have in the bank, what happened in your job or career, what you were able to contribute to yourself, your children and the world-at-large.

Do I have to reiterate that this is meant to be a positive description you create of your life is meant to be a positive description that makes you feel amazing? I hope not, but I just did in case it's necessary for you. Your description is supposed to make you feel amazing as you create it, and every time you think about it.

Be sure to add what you've modeled for your children during your years as their parent. Years ago, I bought the book Young Bucks: How to Raise a Future Millionaire by Troy Dunn after I saw the author on The Big Idea with Donny Deutsch (a great show that sadly, is no longer on the air). Just recently, my budding entrepreneur, a.k.a. my daughter Lexi, brought me the book and asked me to read it with her. The book covers myths about what it takes to become a millionaire. In essence, the book urges parents to foster our children's innate enthusiasm and desire for success. I completely agree with his position. While you're crafting your life-in-review, be sure to envision yourself giving your children the beliefs and encouragement they need to create the life they want to create, too.

The Beginning

There are smart, necessary, and immediate decisions you need to make. For starters, get real about your reality. Things have changed: you may have exited your marriage or relationship with a stash of cash and a good beginning to your future – or not. In either case, it's critically important for you to take stock of where you are versus where you want to end up, and make intelligent, thought-out decisions in that direction.

If you are saddled with debt or don't have an emergency fund, those are your first areas of focus. Every single aspect of your financial life must be uncovered and known. Very simply, you can't get where you want to go (Point B), if you don't know where you are today (Point A).

Clarity and Your Bottom Line

Pull out all of your financial documents and create your Personal Net Worth sheet (you can Google "Personal Net Worth Calculator" and find many simple, easy-to-use forms).

- Make a list of your income sources and amounts.

- Using all of your statements (below), make a list of what you owe (liabilities) and what you have (assets).

- Bank, credit card, and mortgage statements

- Car, student, and personal loans

- Savings and investment account statements

- Make a list of your monthly expenditures, including housing, utilities, groceries, automobile gas and expenditures, education and child care expenses, and so forth. One of the easiest ways to double check that you have included all your monthly expenditures is to look at your check book (bank statement) for the past couple of months. I would recommend you do this for the past year if you have the ability. There may be items like gym memberships, gifts, back to school shopping, and other items that you only pay once in awhile or are due annually that you may want to take into consideration.

Just taking these basic steps will at once help you to obtain clarity and eliminate any resistance you have to knowing where you stand in the big picture. I won't say, "Don't worry," especially if your circumstances seem dire. What I will say is, "It is what it is." You'll now do what you can do to take yourself to the next level, then the next, and then the next.

All you can do is all you really can do, right?

Right!

You know your bottom line and now you can move forward in the future clearly, with no clouds to ruin the view.

Long-term, Intentional Decisions

Just as with any major life-changing event, it's best to wait a year after a divorce or end of a relationship before making any major decisions. Allow no external pressure to cause you to make a move before you're back on your feet emotionally. Until you feel steady and strong, just hang tight. Pay the necessary, immediate bills and do what you must do. Other than that, your job then is to take care of yourself and your kids. The rest can wait.

Once you've taken stock of where you are, you can ask yourself discovery questions to determine what you want to happen next.

- Can you stay in your current home, or do you need or want to move?

- What are some ways to increase your income, or even create additional streams of income?

- Do you need additional education?

- What are your long-term savings, investment, and retirement goals?

These are somewhat surface decisions because ultimately you'll assemble a team that will guide you through the intricacies of your planning, based upon your personal goals and circumstances.

Take Responsibility

If you were the bill payer in the family before, or you've never paid a bill in your life, it's time to take full fiscal responsibility for everything that happens from this day forward.

There are six basic skills you need to have: how to earn more, keep more, spend less than you make, manage and eliminate debt, save intentionally, and invest intelligently.

Did your head just explode? Like I said before, I created my success without ever taking a basic accounting class. Pretty much everything I've learned in my life after my secondary education, I've learned by reading and finding what I needed to know on the Internet.

I learned how to do a mail merge on Microsoft Word by reading about it in the Help section. I learned how to French braid my daughter's hair by following instructions in a book and watching a few YouTube videos. I learned about success by reading about a thousand books in the past twenty-two years.

My point is that you can do anything you set your mind to. You don't need a big, fancy education (but hey, if you've got one or can get one, get after it – i.e., go for it!). But you simply don't need it, you can find out everything you need to know because someone, somewhere has documented a step-by-step process for just about anything, including finances.

This includes learning about finances, your finances. I learned the basics from two keys books: The Richest Man in Babylon and Personal Finance for Dummies. I read both more than fifteen years ago and they changed my life. I learned about tithing, saving, and the basics of investing all at the same time, and I still use those basic principles today: I give away a portion of my income to demonstrate to my subconscious mind there's always an abundance; I have saved (and continue to save) 10% of my income until I eventually accumulated a war-chest to back me up during any unforeseen or unfortunate circumstances; and I invest a portion of my income in my continuing education and self-care.

You get to decide what percentage of what goes where, based upon your long-term goals and objectives, but first, you must …

Systematize and Get Organized!

I'm most happy on Mondays at 6:30 p.m. when my housekeepers leave. Every inch of my house is clean, and every thing is in its place. I feel clear-headed because everything is organized, however, before I could get organized, I had to step back and create systems that would get me there.

Knowing where your key documents are will come in handy when you need them. I had to process a name change this morning and I needed to fax my Marriage Certificate right away. The good news is that I knew exactly where it was and I was able to complete the task in about three minutes.

Just to be clear, the "old Honorée" was a mess! Years ago, the only time I cleaned up was when someone was coming over, not because I was going to be home. I just didn't value myself or my environment enough to keep my home clean and organized, "just" for me. So, if you're not as clean and organized as you'd like to be, don't worry. Your life, your environment, or anything else you want, can change, and you can change them! It all starts with the decision that you are worth it, and then taking consistent, small steps in the direction of becoming more of what you want, such as being more organized, or better with your finances.

Organizing your documents, statements, bills and invoices is easy. You'll need a few items: an expandable file with a pocket for each month, a "to pay" file, and, if you desire and can afford it, a basic accounting software system, like QuickBooks.

In the age of digital everything, I simply scan my important documents, receipts and invoices into my computer and use those files to help my bookkeeper and CPA do their jobs.

When a bill comes, pay it immediately and file it away. If there are bills you cannot pay in full yet, put them in the "to pay" file and pay what you can as soon as you can. Start fresh and clean, neat and organized, as soon as you can and at the beginning of every month thereafter.

As a coach, another system I'll recommend is that you schedule time every month to clean up and organize your documents. Put a reoccurring appointment on your calendar so you won't have to think about it until it's time to think about it, nor will you forget and fall behind, either.

Hold Your Ex Accountable for His Part

This I freely admit was a mistake I made. I got to a point where I was making more than enough money to support myself and my daughter and I stopped holding my ex accountable for his half of Lexi's additional expenses. He always paid child support, but gave me a hard time about any additional bills. Eventually figured I needed my peace of mind more than I needed reimbursement. He's paying now, but he had about five years of not paying for glasses, and for dental, doctor, and therapy visits, to the tune of about $30,000 over the course of those several years.

His first ex-wife always made sure he paid his fair share after their divorce. I didn't always align and agree with her and tried handling the situation my way, which didn't just cost me, it cost my daughter. That is money she won't ever have access to or inherit. Had I thought about having him pay his fair share that way, I would have been more adamant about him paying his fair share.

Yes, you are capable of supporting your kids all on your own. Dealing with an ex can be a huge hassle, emotionally draining, and a general massive pain in the ass. Getting him to pay his share is not about revenge (it shouldn't be, ever); it's about getting what the kids should get. Making sure he pays his share is worth the effort, as everything about our kids is, because taking care of our kids is about taking care of our kids. He's their dad and he should be responsible for his portion of their expenses and upbringing, just as you are their mom and should pay your fair share.

If your ex isn't paying child support, you need to handle that issue, and handle it right away. Use an attorney if you can, but you can take care of it on your own. You can file a motion for contempt of court. He'll have to answer to the Court and explain why he hasn't been compliant. If he's found to be in contempt, there are all sorts of consequences any person would probably want to avoid: asset seizure, fines, even jail. Taking him to court should get you back on the right track, and put the money you need to support your children where it belongs: with you.

If you've got a deadbeat dad on your hands, you can locate him through his motor vehicle, county tax, or personal income tax records. You can also ask city or county social workers to get his mortgage and some banking records, which will help determine his assets and his child support obligation.

Your children deserve to have their father's financial and emotional support, and the law agrees. It took two parents to create the kids and it takes two, ideally, to raise them emotionally and fiscally. You child deserves everything both parents can afford for them and they so richly deserve.

Having a strong financial situation makes you a better relationship seeker and partner.

You may wish to embark on a new love at some point, and it is important to make new relationship decisions from a place of power and not fear. If you're feeling like you just need someone else's income to keep the lights on and food in the fridge, you're more likely to settle for who you get or crosses your path, than if you have a budding war chest. Financial stability is one crucial piece of the puzzle to ensure you make your relationship decisions from a place of "want to" not "have to."

With any new relationship, you'll want to ensure that your personal financial style is in alignment or complimentary to your mate's, just as ensure your spiritual, religious and even parenting styles are in alignment or complimentary.

After I got divorced, my therapist recommended that I not embark on a new relationship for at least two years. She said it took one year to heal, and a second year to discover my new self. I thought two years sounded like forever, internally disagreed with her, and thought I knew better. Well, I didn't. It did take just about two years to feel like myself again and feel ready to start a new relationship. In those two years, I made some big mistakes I regret, a few of them financial ones. Be sure you have a support system, even if they're paid, to help you navigate making any financial decisions with a new love. Make sure you're protected whenever you make those moves, especially if you have assets you want to hold on to.

CHAPTER THREE

DEFINING RICH, FOR YOU

*"Keep your feet on the ground and your thoughts
at lofty heights."* ~Peace Pilgrim

Why Setting Goals is Critical

There is power in precision. Setting goals is important
to success, and you are worthy of creating and having
success. It's truly remarkable what people can accomplish
when they focus their energy and attention on achieving
something they really want to achieve. Set correctly, your
goals get you out of bed before your alarm sounds in the
morning and keep you up late at night ... not that as single
moms, we're getting much sleep anyway. However, when
goals instead of stress and worry are keeping you up, that's
just better!

What Do YOU Want?

As I've said previously, rich means different things to

different people … and however you define rich is fine, no matter how much or how little actual money is involved. To me, I know you'll be rich when you have more than enough money to support yourself and your kids in your desired lifestyle, and you feel amazing about yourself and your situation.

Setting your goals based on your wants and desires will propel you forward and get you where you want to be faster, easier, and with less effort.

Let me expand on goals just a bit. Based on the areas you focused on in your vision, the next step is to identify goals based on that vision. Here are some ideas to help you get started.

Coach's Commandments for Goal-Setting:

1. Write down your goals. This step is the most important aspect of goal setting. Writing down your goals creates the roadmap to your success.

Coach's Insight: Although just the act of writing them down can set the process in motion, it's also extremely important to review your goals frequently. Remember, the more focused you are on your goals, the more likely you are to accomplish them.

Sometimes we realize we have to revise a goal because circumstances and other goals change. If you need to change a goal, don't consider changing a goal a failure. Instead, consider it a victory because you had the insight to realize the goal you set wasn't perfect, and you had the courage to make a change!

"Write it down. Written goals have a way of transforming wishes into wants; cant's into cans,

dreams into plans, and plans into reality.
Don't just think it -- ink it!" ~Author Unknown

"If you don't see it, you will never be it."
~Author Known (me)

2. Your goals should be based solely on your vision.

Based on the vision you have for yourself, setting tangible goals is the next critical step. Write your goals in positive language. Define and work for what you want, not what you want to leave behind. You are using language to focus your brain in the exact direction you want it to take you. Part of the reason for writing down, examining and re-examining your goals is to create a set of instructions for your subconscious mind to carry out. Your subconscious mind is an efficient, powerful tool that does not distinguish the real from the imagined, and it does not judge. It's only function is to carry out instructions. The more positive instructions you give it, the more positive results you will get, and the faster you will get them.

3. Make your goals congruent with each other.

In other words, one goal must not contradict any of your other goals.

A goal to buy a $750,000 home is incongruent with an income goal of $50,000 per year. This is called non-integrated thinking and will sabotage all of the hard work you put into your goals. Non-integrated thinking can also hamper your everyday thoughts as well.

4. Make your goals specific, precise, and clearly defined.

Just like your vision, write out your goals in complete, vivid detail! Instead of writing "a new home," describe the home you desire: "A 7,500 square foot contemporary with 5 bedrooms, 3 baths, an office with a separate entrance, and a view of the mountains on 20 acres of land."

Once again, giving the subconscious mind a detailed set of instructions is crucial to goal achievement. The clearer you are, and the more specific information you give the subconscious mind, the clearer the final outcome becomes, and the more efficiently the subconscious mind works to turn your dreams into reality.

Can you close your eyes and visualize the home I described above? Walk around the house. Stand on the porch off the master bedroom and see the fog lifting off the mountains. Look down at the garden full of tomatoes, green beans, and cucumbers. Off to the right is another garden full of mums, carnations and roses. Can you see it? So can your subconscious mind, and it will work relentlessly to bring your vision to reality as quickly as possible, and in the exact way you have imagined.

This area is where your mind has worked "for you" but seemingly against you in the past. It has created what you have previously held in your mind as your vision. This is another reason to have a clearly defined, written vision of your desired future.

5. Include a timeline.

Timelines are vital to goal achievement. Exactly when must this goal be achieved? "This year," "soon," "in a little while," or "later" doesn't cut it. Pick a date. If what you want is not on the calendar, it's not going to happen. Your timeline will need to be written in the following format, "By June 30th, I have 12 new customers who purchase my services at $2,500 each." You must be able to measure exactly where you stand now against where you want to be in the future.

"A goal is a dream with a deadline." ~Napoleon Hill

6. Make sure your goals are big enough!

I'm sure you've heard the old saying, "Shoot for the moon. If you miss, you'll still reach the stars." Goals should inspire you to move forward, perhaps with a little bit of a knot in your stomach. If your goals are too easy, you won't be as motivated to achieve them. If they're too hard, you might become overwhelmed and not even take the first, necessary steps.

Set your goals now. (Is there going to be a better time?) Pull out your journal and set four goals you would like to achieve in the next year. Taking action right away reinforces to your subconscious mind you are serious about achieving your vision.

What's Next?

I recommend that you keep your goals to yourself. Share them only with those people you absolutely, 100% know will support and encourage you. Stay away from "dream stealers." Negative attitudes from friends and family can drag you down at the speed of sound. It's critical that your self-talk, the thoughts in your head, and the talk around you are positive.

Reviewing your goals daily is crucial to your success and must become part of your routine.

Make copies to put in different places in your office, car and home to keep you on track. I post my goals everywhere – above my treadmill, on my bathroom mirror, on my desk, in my car. In every possible moment, I want to be reminded of what I want to have, do, be and create.

Each morning when you wake up, read your list of goals. Spend a few moments visualizing each goal as completed: see your new completely furnished home, smell the leather seats in your hot new sports car, feel the cold hard cash in your hands (or, in my case, using my MasterCard at Nordstrom's ... often). Visualize yourself on that vacation to sunny Mexico, the sun warm on your skin as you sip piña coladas beside the clear blue ocean. Vividly picturing your goals completed triggers your brain to move you automatically toward your vision as quickly as possible.

Each night just before bed, repeat the process. This will start both your conscious and subconscious mind working towards your goals. Replace any negative self-talk and images with the positive energy you need to move forward.

Every time you make a decision or take an action during the day, ask yourself: "Does this take me closer to or farther away from, my goal?" If the answer is "closer to," then you've made the right decision. If the answer is "farther from," well ... you know what to do!

Follow this process everyday, and you'll be on your way to achieving unlimited success in every aspect of your life.

Your Long-term Goals

Because you've created a vision of your future, you're in the habit of writing things down, and you have the how-to's for goal setting, you can probably create your long-term goals pretty quickly. One goal might be to retire once you have $1,000,000 in the bank and your home is paid in full. Another might be to buy a home within two years, and save $25,000 toward a down payment.

I have a goal for how much I want to give to non-profits and charities. It's a number that is a percentage of my overall income. Once I've achieved that goal I will have given a lot, which means I've made a lot. That's one way I keep myself focused and moving forward.

If you have not written down your goals already, be sure to schedule an hour to pull out your journal and ink those goals!

Your Short-term Goals

Unfortunately, retirement or even two years is a long time away. You'll need instant and on-going motivation to keep you moving forward and focused.

If you don't have shorter-term goals, you will give in to impulse purchases, not giving a second thought to buying those on-sale boots or jetting off for a weekend.

I am an avid watcher of <u>The Nate Berkus Show</u>. He regularly does segments on buying more with less, do-it-yourself projects, and how to be better with money. Recently, he interviewed a woman recently who paid off almost $24,000 in debt over fourteen months. She had a short-term goal and took no prisoners in achieving it! Your short-term goals weave the cloth for those long-term goals to be achieved, so set some short-term goals about two seconds after you've set your long-term goals.

I believe that "having an emergency fund" should be goal number one. If you don't have at least three months of living expenses in a savings account you can access at any time, an emergency fund is a great place to start. Another great starter goal is to get rid of any debt you may have. I've been in debt and I absolutely hate it. I now refuse to buy anything I can't pay for in cash, and won't take on any "bad" debt. There's more detail on "bad" versus "good" debt coming up, I've got a whole chapter on debt to help you manage and get out of yours.

One more perfect short-term initial goal is "to start saving 10%" or whatever percent you can start with. I had a friend who was heavily in debt, under-water on her mortgage and barely making ends meet. So, she started with 1%. Later, as her savings grew and grew, she described saving as an obsession! She loved making those transfers into her savings account and had lots of fun calculating how much would be there in a year, five years, ten years and "someday." She's also so much more relaxed, now that she has a reserve.

Remember this: the best time to have started something was five or ten years ago. The next best time to start something is right now. If you haven't started paying off your debt or saving money, you can literally start right now. It takes moments to open a checking account online and usually about $25. Raid the sugar bowl or couch cushions if you have to and do it today. You'll be so exceedingly glad you did.

Making Positive Progress: Track It to Max It

What you give your attention to will expand. If you want maximum results, you must regularly check in and track your progress. It's like getting on the scale once a year, if you don't know what's happening on a pretty regular basis, anything can happen and usually does.

It is important to figure out a tracking system that works for you. You can create your own Excel spreadsheet, use a simple notebook, or go high-tech and log everything (for free) at a website like Mint.com or use Quicken Free Personal Finance Software. Both have tons of resources for you to guide you on your path. Whatever system you choose, you will be executing such an important step toward your future riches.

CHAPTER FOUR

DO YOU SPEAK MONEY?

"Form the habit of thinking and talking prosperity and abundance, and soon prosperity and abundance will become your reality." ~Honorée Corder

Here's a language you need to speak is money! Forgive me if I'm covering a subject about which you have more knowledge than I do. There was a time when I was learning even the most basic of concepts, and I want to include them here just in case even one of my single mom readers needs them.

Learning something new can be challenging and overwhelming. I'm going to give you the basics, introduce you to the future members of your financial team, and they can take it from there.

If you don't have this basic knowledge, and you run into someone who doesn't have the best of intentions, you can make mistakes that would have been avoidable.

Full disclosure: I'm not a financial advisor, attorney, CPA or bookkeeper, but I have my own team and I find them invaluable. I didn't need a team when I had debt, a non-profitable business, and no assets. However, as I've grown, so has my desire and need to have the professionals on standby who know what to do with someone in my situation. As you progress on your financial journey, you'll want to find the same professionals to help you, too.

Your Homework

First, you've got to learn the lingo: the very least you need to know. Then, you need to enroll yourself in a self-learning program where you seek out new information so you can make informed, educated decisions. At first, you'll make these decisions on your own, but eventually you'll discuss your options with your team.

Basic Financial Vocabulary

Your Monthly Nut: you may refer to it as your budget. I personally don't like the word budget because to me it's limiting. and it's kind of like the term step-mother. It just doesn't have a good feeling about it. Your monthly nut is a comprehensive list of your monthly expenses. In other words, how much does it take for you to keep your current lifestyle fully paid for without incurring debt or borrowing from your savings? For right now, this is everything on your Personal Net Worth Calculator.

Assets: This term refers to how much you own, have saved, have in investments, including valuables, property, businesses and monies owed to you.

Liabilities: Everything you owe: mortgages, car loans, student loans, personal loans, credit card debt, etc. If you owe it, it's a liability.

Net Worth: Subtract your liabilities from your assets and that is your net worth.

What if your number is negative? Well, then zero is the first goal: to owe nothing and be on the way to having a positive number in the assets category.

We'll talk about this topic more in the chapter on debt.

Needs vs. Wants

I know this is a silly question, but do you know the difference? Of course you do. Does the difference really matter? In my opinion, no.

I believe we live in an abundant universe and that if you truly want something, you can have it. Of course you would probably be best served by taking care of your needs first. Having a place to live, clothes to wear, food to eat, and something to get around in would be most helpful. We are able, I believe, to have whatever we truly want, therefore, I'm not going to advise you to create a strict budget (again, I dislike that word), go without, have a home that's too warm in the summer and too cold in the winter to save a few pennies.

Hopefully, I'm going to help you to expand into the life you'd truly like to live.

Of course, I also believe in hard work, acting prudently and intelligently, and doing every action with intention.

My Philosophy On Saving and Investing (The Basics)

When I read *The Richest Man in Babylon* and *Personal Finance for Dummies* I learned to tithe, which is giving a portion of one's income back to their source of spiritual nourishment. I also learned to pay myself first by saving 10% of my income until I had at least three months worth of living expenses in the bank. Once I hit that benchmark, I could then begin to invest based upon my risk tolerance.

I read something quite interesting in my early twenties, and that was this: if you save 10% of your income between the age of 20 and 30, it would be the same with compounded interest as saving between age 30 and 65. Ten years versus thirty-five years. Wow!

That possibility really hit home for me, and ever since then I have told everyone in their twenties to just do themselves a favor and get in the habit of saving.

When I receive any kind of income, including payment for services or products, royalties from books or licensing, or when random strangers walk up to me and hand me a wad of cash, I do two things: I tithe ten percent and I save ten percent.

Note: Random strangers don't walk up to me and hand me wads of cash, but I'm keeping an open mind so I'm ready when they are!

There have been many times when I haven't had enough cash on hand to handle a situation, so I've dipped into my savings (and I always pay myself back as soon as I can), but I don't have to use credit cards or credit lines. I can loan myself money, thereby eliminating paying interest and finance charges. I operate under the "pay as I go" principles, which also precludes me from having buyers remorse.

How much, then, do you need? I'll be exploring with you many options for creating more income. For right now, it's about how much you need on a monthly basis. Based upon your monthly nut, you may <u>need</u> $5,000. In my world, that means you need to make $7,500. I like to multiply everything by 150%. If $5,000 pays the bills, that's nothing for giving back, for saving, or fun, or for challenges. In truth, you need $7,500 so you can have money for giving back (10% equals $500), and saving (10% equals $500), or fun, or challenges (you've still got $1,500 for these).

What if your car breaks down, you need a new pair of shoes, and your kid takes up playing the clarinet and needs an instrument and other paraphernalia? Or, you have the opportunity to attend someone's wedding or birthday party? If you don't have an abundance of funds, there's no abundance of fun!

Build into your personal financial goals money to give back, save for yourself and your future, and to have some fun. Trust me when I say there is supply for your new demand. Money you need will show up! More on that subject in Chapter 9, Creating Wealth, Mind over Manifesting.

Once you've built up some reserves, you'll need to begin to assemble your Dream Team.

Why Having a Dream Team is Important

I chose the term "Dream Team" on purpose because having the right people on your Dream Team can help make your dreams a reality, and much more quickly than you could do it on your own.

I think it's imperative for you to do as much of the work as possible, rather than turning control over to someone else. Having the knowledge you need to make intelligent decisions is important and you are smart enough to learn everything you need to learn. You can't do it alone, but let's cut to the chase here: what happens to your money affects the quality of your life, not the life of your financial advisor, banker, or insurance agent's. Just your life. It's essential, therefore, that you understand what is going on, and are able to make informed decisions for yourself. In fact, I am convinced you have what it takes to go it alone, especially with the easy-to-follow guide I am here to give you on the key steps you need to take to manage your finances.

If you're employed or have just started a business, you'll need a banker, insurance agent, and financial advisor.

Your Personal and Business Banker

Starting with your basic banking options, here are a few techniques and tips for being successful in locating a good bank and a great banker.

1.   Never pick a bank, always pick a banker. The individual you work with is usually more important than the institution you choose.

2.   The best way to find a good banker is to ask for a referral from a mentor or successful entrepreneur.

3.   After you have a banker, make them familiar with your situation and issues. They can be instrumental in helping you to have the right kinds of accounts, as well as secure funding if and when the time comes.

Financial Advisor

Just like with your banker, you're going to want to know, like and trust your financial advisor. I believe first impressions are important, so here are a few qualities to look for:

- Someone who has you come to his or her office. If he or she comes to you, it's a sign they have too much time on their hands.

- A good financial planner will ask good questions, for the planner's job is to truly understand the total financial situation of your household, which means he or she should want to be familiar with your needs, wants, and risks.

- Does he or she have a clean office and desk? A planner who isn't organized isn't the right person to handle your money.

- You want a planner who works on a "fee-only" basis. Advisers should not make a penny off of commissions from investments they recommend you make. You can't trust someone who makes their living based on how often you buy and sell investments.

As for the actual interview, when you are talking to a planner you'll want to keep track of what is being covered. From the start, keep an ear out for a prospective adviser who immediately launches into stocks or mutual funds you should buy, they are someone you should run from. Investing is just a small part of your financial needs, and besides, how can a person know what you should buy before they know anything about you? Before a planner tells you what to invest in, they should have talked to you about:

- Your overall situation and your goals for the

future.

- The importance of a Will and Living Revocable Trust.

- Whether you have any debt other than a mortgage, such as credit card debt, student loan debt, and so forth.

- Your FICO (credit) score and how it will impact your financial moves.

- Whether you anticipate needing to provide financial assistance to your parents during their retirement, and/or receiving an inheritance from them.

- Your plans for a family, especially whether you intend to send your children to private school and to what extent you intend to finance their college education.

- Whether you rent or own a home, and what your goals in this area are. Do you want to trade up to a bigger place or different neighborhood, or do you want to downsize?

- Your life insurance needs, because you have others dependent on your income.

- Retirement investments you already have, such as 401(k)s and IRAs.

- What you want to achieve with your

investments: what your investment horizon is (Five years? Ten years? Thirty?) and how much risk you are comfortable with, meaning can you handle your portfolio falling, say, 15 percent so you can stay in position to reap potential gains over the longer term?

Insurance Agent

I consulted my agent, Fred Bangasser, with New York Life, for his input on selecting the right agent. Fred advised that as a single mom, you want to make absolute certain you select the "right agent." Ask some of your trusted friends for recommendations. Interview several agents and select one who has (most of) the following qualities:

a. You can meet on a friendly basis and feel he or she is competent. Remember that your agent will be working with your loved ones in the event something happens to you.

b. Has professional designations (CLU, ChFC, CFP, MBA, etc.,) and is a member of the Million Dollar Round Table (MDRT), thereby showing their experience and dedication to the insurance industry.

c. He or she has been in the business for more than five years. Many agents drop out of the business in their early years. You want someone with experience to serve you.

When you purchase insurance, you want to select a company that has:

a. Top ratings from the four different rating officials (A.M. Best, Standard and Poor's, Moody's and Fitch).

b. Been around for more than 50 years.

    c.   A mutual-fund company vs. a stock company.

Finally, Fred offered this gem: "Cheap things are of no value, and valuable things are not cheap." Insurance lasts a lifetime. You want a company to be there on the day you die to pay the claim.

He also recommends that if you haven't completed your divorce, that part of the divorce settlement includes both a life and a disability policy taken out to cover any child support arrangements and college expenses. The policy should be taken out on the person who is to pay the support payments, but owned by the person receiving the benefits. Therefore, any changes to the policy contracts (or failure to pay premiums when due) will be immediately known by the proper person. If you've already completed your divorce settlement, it's a good idea to broach the subject if at all possible.

Certified Public Accountant (CPA)

Taxpayers of all types can benefit from hiring a tax accountant, but before you spend your hard-earned cash, here's some simple steps you can take to protect yourself, to find the right professional for your situation, and some questions to ask.

Understand Why You Need a Tax Accountant

You should take some time to focus on exactly what you need your tax accountant to do. Here are some common situations:

- Preparing your own taxes is time-consuming, stressful, or confusing.

- You want to make sure your tax returns are accurate.

- Your tax situation is pretty complex, and you need specialized advice and tips.

- You would like to pay as little taxes as possible and need detailed planning and advice.

- You are facing a tax problem, such as filing back taxes, paying off a tax debt, or fighting an IRS audit.

- You run a business, invest in the stock market, own rental property, or live outside the United States.

Finding the Right Tax Accountant

You should find an experienced tax accountant who specializes in the areas you need help with. Here are my tips for finding the right professional who has the specialized tax expertise you need:

- Referrals are your best bet. Ask everyone you can think of: family, friends, business owners, financial advisors and attorneys. It will help to ask someone who has a similar tax situation to yours.

- Be wary of an accountant who promises you big refunds or that says you can deduct everything. You, not the accountant, are ultimately responsible for the information on your tax return.

- Do not be afraid to shop around or to change

accountants if you are not comfortable.

•   Retail tax franchises such as H&R Block, Jackson Hewitt, and Liberty Tax Service offer competent tax service for individuals who need to file relatively straight-forward tax returns. Some tax preparers will be more experienced than others, and you can sometimes find CPAs and Enrolled Agents working in these offices. Prices are often determined by how many tax forms need to be filled out. Here's a tip: ask if you can meet with a CPA, enrolled agent, or senior tax preparer. You'll pay the same, but you'll get to speak with a seasoned professional.

•   Local, independent tax firms often specialize in the tax needs of individuals and small businesses in their neighborhood. Again, some independent tax accountants will be more experienced than others. Ask if the firm has the expertise to handle your taxes.

•   Enrolled Agents (EAs) are tax professionals who have passed a rigorous test and background check administered by the IRS. Enrolled agents often specialize and are best for complex tax situations.

•   Certified Public Accountants (CPAs) are accountants who have passed the rigorous CPA Exam and are licensed by the state in which they work. CPAs will specialize in a specific area, such as audits, tax, or business consulting. CPAs are best at complex accounting work, but not all CPAs handle tax issues.

• Tax attorneys are lawyers who have chosen to specialize in tax law. Often, tax attorneys will have a master of law degree in taxation (LL.M.) in addition to the required juris doctor (J.D.) degree. Attorneys are best at complex legal matters, such as preparing estate tax returns or taking your case before the US Tax Court.

• Certain CPAs can also be excellent financial advisors. The CPAs in your town generally have their hands around the business community and can be a great source of referrals. They can help you prepare financial statements, point you in the right direction for loans (business or personal), and help you plan out your life. They generally have a wealth of knowledge and understand the big picture of your community. Be wary of the CPA that wants to personally sell you insurance or direct you to purchase certain annuities, stocks or mutual funds.

Questions to Ask an Accountant

The tax industry is constantly changing and tax professionals are subject to various federal and state regulations. Here are some questions you can ask to help ensure you find an experienced, trustworthy tax accountant:

• What licenses or designations do you have?

• How long have you been in the tax business?

• What tax issues do you specialize in?

- Do you have the knowledge and experience to handle my tax situation?

- What are your fees?

- Do you outsource any of your work? Do you perform the work personally? If not, what is the review process? Who signs the returns?

- How long, approximately, will it take to finish my taxes?

- What's your privacy policy? Will you share my tax information with any third-parties?

- Do you believe I'm paying too much, too little, or just the right amount of tax?

- Can you advise me if I change my circumstances (marry, start a business, have another child)?

Tax accountants come from a wide variety of backgrounds, and have different attitudes about our tax system (in the United States). The idea is that you should find an experienced, competent tax accountant who specializes in the areas you need help with, and someone who believes in helping you to minimize your taxes.

After your interview, you'll want to perform a quick background check. Contact your state's board of accountancy to check the status of a CPA's license, or to find out if any disciplinary action has been taken against the CPA. For enrolled agents, you can ask the IRS Office of Professional Responsibility if an EA has been censured, disbarred or subjected to other disciplinary action.

Successful Single Mom Julie Booth's Story

In her own words, Julie shared what's happened since she was featured in The Successful Single Mom book.

"I am finally at a point in my life where I can say I am at ease. I am able to drop my daughter, Hannah, off at school in the morning and pick her up when school ends at 3:00pm. I wasn't even able to do that when I was married! I am able to talk to other moms and her teacher after school. I am dialed into my daughter's life and more connected. I am able to show up to Parent/Teacher conferences in the middle of the day and pick Hannah up from school when she is sick. I am able to help at school events, and even schedule some time to help the teacher during the day. I don't have that panicked feeling when something upsets my daily routine. If I am in a meeting at a client's office and get the dreaded call from school (we all know that call and feeling when we are at work), I have three awesome moms on my street that I can call to back me up.

I am a strong believer in spending the time to get a network or team of people behind you as a single mom. I know for some moms that is a scary issue, it sure was for me, but I am truly reaping the benefits today for stepping outside of my comfort zone. I walk every morning at 5 a.m. with two other moms on my street. We walk for an hour and we talk about everything. It is a great way to start my day, and I have actually gained a couple clients by listening to their needs and answering some questions, because they referred me to a couple people. I don't think single or even married moms understand how much we need each other. The two moms I walk with in the morning are both married and have completely accepted me into the group. I used to have the "stigma," the feeling that married moms would never understand, help, or befriend me. I was amazed when I found that one of the moms was divorced in the past and had blended her current family. My fear was the only thing holding me back. I now have an awesome friend who has already been through my same situation, can mentor me and answer my questions.

The biggest thing that has helped me since getting divorced January 2007 is setting boundaries. They have helped me take my power back. I know they are not easy, and I am the first to admit that I am not 100% successful with my boundaries. However, the boundaries have allowed me to obtain and retain a successful relationship with an awesome man. Having quality friends and a support team has helped me tackle the tough phase of introducing Hannah to a man. I remained single for 2 years after separating from Hannah's dad because I needed to get my life together and in order. During that time, I followed the "Successful Single Mom" 100-day plan, found myself and what I really wanted in life. I think all moms and dads would benefit from the "Successful Single Mom" plan that Honorée has created! I am very happy I took the time to follow through, and today am reaping the benefits for believing in myself. Every mom has the ability, knowledge and creativity within her. It is just a matter of doing it, and you can do it, too!"

Estate Planning Attorney

Your estate plan will eventually have a profound effect on your loved ones' lives and well-being. You should spend time and effort searching for the right estate-planning attorney, because the right one can help you pass on your riches, wealth, and abundance in the spirit in which you want it disbursed. If you are a first-generation wealth accumulator, do some reading about what happens when the second generation gets its hands on the money! You may wish, as I do, to pass on wealth with values attached, and the right estate planning attorney will help you to distribute your wealth with clauses that protect the wealth and the recipients.

I consulted Darci Poloni, who is both a successful single mom and an estate-planning attorney. Darci has been practicing law for 15 years, and is the Managing Partner of her own firm, Poloni & Associates, P.C., located in Henderson, Nevada. Her practice focuses exclusively on estate planning and corporate law. She is a graduate of the University of Southern California Law School. She has lived and practiced estate planning in the Las Vegas Valley since 2003. All of that, and she is a single mom with a beautiful five-year old daughter.

Here's her advice for you:

"Single Moms, in particular, should not forget about estate planning. Estate planning is the process of identifying who you would like to raise your children if you pass away or become incapacitated, who you would like to handle your finances if you cannot, who will enforce your end of life health care decisions, and who will specify what those decisions are concerning how and when you want your assets distributed to your heirs (yes, you can put conditions on your child's inheritance). Most estate plans include a revocable living trust, a pour-over will, health care and financial powers of attorney and funding documents. Estate planning is also an effective tool to avoid the costly and lengthy probate process in most states.

When interviewing estate-planning attorneys, consider whether the lawyer specializes or dabbles in estate planning. You don't want to hire an attorney who was a bankruptcy specialist a month ago and a personal injury attorney the month before that. Estate and tax laws change frequently. It's crucial that the attorney you select specializes in this area and is committed to staying abreast of all changes in the law affecting your estate plan. Be careful of "estate planning attorneys" that only go half way or just draft your legal documents. They will set up your living trust but tell you that it's your obligation to "fund" it. These lawyers are counting on the fact that you will be so overwhelmed by the funding process that you will fail to do it (or only complete a portion of the funding), and then when you pass away, they will handle the probate process for your family, thereby earning double fees. Simply put, your trust does nothing for you unless it is fully funded. All of your assets must be transferred to your trust.

There are some exceptions; however, such as retirement plans, which may have negative tax consequences of being funded in your trust, which is another reason that I strongly recommend that you hire a knowledgeable estate-planning attorney that has been in practice for some time and has no intention of retiring any time soon. Of course, personality is also a key factor in selecting an attorney. This is a sensitive time in which you will make very serious decisions regarding the end of your life. I urge you to make sure that you are comfortable with your attorney and that you believe he or she has your best interests in mind."

Your Personal Coach

World-class athletes, CEOs of major corporations and winners in nearly every profession know that without a coach, the right coach, they won't perform at their peak. With the right coach, the sky is the limit. I absolutely believe everyone needs a coach. Not because I am a coach, but because I have a coach

My first experience with a coach was when I had my Shaklee business: I had achieved a top-level position and was doing everything I thought I needed to do to reach my goals and objectives within the fastest possible time frame. When the CEO of Shaklee called to offer me a business coach, my first thoughts were: "What could I possibly need with a coach? I'm already doing great!" Fortunately, I kept my mouth shut, accepted the incredible gift of a coach, and I'm so glad I did. Within 90 days I had increased my overall productivity and income by 300%. The distinctions I made about myself, the way I was using my time, identifying bigger goals, defining a larger vision and being held accountable were all crucial to me.

My coach was able to see what I wasn't able to see. She helped me to take risks, eliminate obstacles, and step fully into my potential.

A coach's function is multi-faceted: to blend insights, tools and key traits to move clients toward success in many areas, both on the job and off. Performers at all levels are elevated to greater advancement in the presence of an effective coach.

As previously mentioned, the value of coaching is clearly understood in the world of sports. Tiger Woods needs a coach to excel. If the number one golfer in the world relies on the power of coaching, wouldn't anyone in the business world benefit from applying the same principle?

I would venture to guess not a day goes by that Tiger Woods doesn't speak with his "head" coach, or work with his "form" coach to fine-tune his chip shot, drive or putt. Yet many people step into business and leadership positions with little direction, and few goals or strategies for growth and development. Rarely do they seek help acquiring leadership skills or identifying hidden strengths.

Choosing to have a great coach in your corner can accelerate your success. Coaches are not for the meek. They're for people who value unambiguous feedback. The best coaches have one thing in common: they are mercilessly results-oriented. Also, coaching isn't therapy. It's product development, and you are the product.

"Coaching is the means through which we come to realize our greatest potential."
~Ryan C. Browning (my coach)

How to Get the Most Out of Your Coach

Insist on complete confidentiality between the coach and yourself, meaning all conversations are private and sacred. Confidentiality should be part of the coaching agreement you sign. Your coach should not acknowledge you are a client to anyone else unless you give your permission. What you are doing, how you are doing, what you have accomplished, and your personal secrets are not discussed or even hinted at with anyone else. People may know you are working with a coach, and may ask how you are doing. Your coach's standard answer should be: "He/she is doing just fine." (Period.)

Insist on measurable goals. To ensure that your work with a coach doesn't become an exercise in unproductive conversation, tie everything to a business benefit. By itself, "improve time-management skills" has no measurable benefit, but the phrase is a legitimate way to achieve a critical goal, "to meet project deadlines in 30% less time."

Set tangible goals. Now isn't the time for stretch goals, instead aim for improvements that you know you can achieve. Most people aren't working on even half their cylinders. Don't strive for 100% improvement – a 15% improvement is the difference between a mediocre player and a star.

When it comes to assessing your performance, ask your coach to be exhaustively honest with you. Some are not. Take these sound bites of coaches describing their role: "I just hold the CEO's hand," says one. "I'm like a trusted family friend," says another. Or: "My job is to remind him, 'your greatest strength is that you're you.'"

If you get that warm, fuzzy feeling from a coach, run! Look for a coach who isn't afraid to use constructive criticism. Coaches are best when they push you out of your comfort zone, *and don't let you back in.*

Are You Ready for Coaching?

If you're now ready to consider hiring a coach, you are really deciding to embark on a magnificent journey! Coaching is proven to work when two factors are present:

a. The client is willing to grow.

b. There is a gap (or several gaps) between where you are now and where you want to be.

These two criteria are all that's necessary for you and your coach to address and resolve challenges, create new focus and direction, move your life and/or business in the right direction, dramatically increase sales and profitability, as well as devise and execute a plan of action.

Once you've hired your coach, you will enroll in specific programs that can include:

Coaching for skills. The focus on a specific task or skill set, such as making presentations, preparing a business plan, etc.

Coaching for performance. Here, the focus is on improving existing job performance and might involve such things as developing systems to evaluate employee performance accurately.

Coaching for development, involves concentrating on an individual's future career path.

Coaching on a variety of topics. This program recognizes that executives can be lonely and frequently need insight, perspective and constructive feedback on both personal and business issues. It could also include developing specific leadership skills such as emotional intelligence (EQ).

With some great coaching, you will compress the amount of time it takes to reach your goals. You will also have someone who believes in you, holds your vision for you and can keep you moving in just the right direction. I know you will benefit and enjoy having a coach as much as I do.

Childcare

The most critical member of your Dream Team is the person you rely on to take care of your children when they are not in school or with their father. You can hire a professional nanny or governess. You can hire a teenager. You can rely on friends and relatives. You can create a group of single moms who trades favors and childcare. Many hands make light work, and having even just a couple of single mom friends who can help will make a huge difference in both what you're able to get done and your stress level.

With no family and no money, you're left to get creative. I shared my situation in The Successful Single Mom book and how I dealt with my situation. In order to excel in your business or job, have time for yourself and be the best mom you can be, you will need regular breaks from your kids. It's a fact of life that we love them, but we can't spend 24/7 with them.

Brainstorm all of the different ways you can arrange for the care your kids will need while you get done what needs to get done.

I've thrown a lot at you in this chapter. Take a deep breath and know it will always be here to use as a reference. Be deliberate in learning new financial skills, and in choosing your Dream Team. I'm years down the road on this journey, and let me tell you it feels good to have both knowledge and people who can help me be my best in all areas, because I know my financial house is in order. You can make significant progress, starting today, by simply putting one foot in front of the other.

CHAPTER FIVE

IF YOU HAVE DEBT

*"Replace your habit of spending with the
habit of saving and you will attain
financial independence."*
~Honorée Corder

At different times in my life, I've had debt. Not a lot, but enough to be uncomfortable and wishing I didn't have any. Zero was my first goal, and I played both ends to the middle: I paid myself first by putting money into savings while at the same time paying off my debt. I don't think it serves you to just pay off your debt and have no cash reserves for challenges or opportunities. I advise you not to focus on your debt because doesn't focusing on your debt make your blood pressure rise? It does mine!

I'll steal a line from Bob Proctor, a teacher in the book, <u>The Secret</u>: "Set up a debt repayment program and then focus on making more money." While you shouldn't just pretend that your debt doesn't exist, once you've set up a system to eliminate it, there's no sense giving it your attention any longer.

Cash is King, Debt is Detrimental

At this time in the fall of 2011, because of the economy of the past couple of years, there are a ton of opportunities to buy things "on sale" (literally pennies on the dollar) if you have cash, such as businesses and even homes. Having cash reserves gives you a shot at opportunities you won't have if you have to get a loan or borrow on a credit line. Just a few short years ago, real estate, land, cars and gems were going at premium prices. Today, those same items are being off-loaded by folks who aren't as cash-rich or even credit-line-rich as they were before. If you have cash, you can often buy a variety of goodies at a deep discount.

Therefore, while you're paying down your debt, simultaneously be saving, even if you choose to save less and pay off more debt. Your savings will incur interest and you can begin to enjoy the dollars you save compounding, even while you sleep!

If you have developed the habit of incurring debt and you don't rise above it, you will miss out on what's possible for you because debt is like quicksand and the more you move around in it, the further you sink.

Different Kinds Of Debt

There are two types of debt:

- Good debt: the kind you take on to get professional training or education, or invest in something that has a high rate of return. This is the kind of debt that can eventually make you money.

- Bad debt: the kind you take on to purchase luxuries and non-necessary items. This kind of debt costs you money, so no matter what you buy, you are paying more for it than you intended.

When you borrow to educate yourself, you are empowered and very often the interest rates are low because even financial institutions and the government understand the value of education. Avoid bad debt at all costs: you want your "babies making babies" (more on this in a minute), not your dollars borrowed costing you money in fees and interest. Psychologically, debt isn't great either. Bad debt feels like dead weight; it works against your willpower and causes a loss of ambition. It literally sucks the life and positive energy right out of you, and sadly, if you don't stop incurring it, you will probably never be able to dig out of it and restore your lost fortune.

From *Law of Success* by Napoleon Hill:

> *"The person who is free from debt may whip poverty and achieve outstanding financial success, but, if bound by debt, such achievement is only a remote possibility, and never a probability."*

> *I want you to begin to empower yourself by putting the first of many dollars into your eventual war chest. Now, let's get you started on that journey.*

Get Out of Debt Fastest and Cheapest, Get Into Saving

There are a few simple steps you can take to begin to eliminate your debt forever.

- Before you make your next round of payments, call each creditor and ask them to lower your interest rate. You don't ask, you don't get – the banks don't want you to ask for a lower rate and they certainly won't offer it, but if you ask, many times they will lower it, especially if you make them aware you are willing to take your business elsewhere.

• Now, make a list of your debts, and put the highest interest balance at the top.

• Pay the minimum payment for each balance with the exception of the first one: pay the minimum payment with an additional $5, or more if you can swing it.

• Pay off the highest interest rate balance and once it's gone, continue to pay the same amount, just allocate the money to the other debts and watch them quickly disappear.

• Some credit card companies have added to their statements a recommendation for a payment you can make if you want to get out of debt in three or five years. If you can make that payment, make it.

You do have another option, if paying the debt has become a true hardship. If making just the minimum payments is so overwhelming you're not meeting your basic needs without a huge level of stress, you can call each of your creditors and ask them to settle the debt with you. As long as you're current with your payments, they won't work with you, but if you fall behind or have fallen behind, often they will freeze the interest and allow you to pay down just the principle, lower your payments, and extend the amount of time you have to pay. Sometimes they will take a lump sum that is a fraction of the total owed.

While there are many third-party programs available, they all charge a large fee and the work they do is work you can do yourself. It's up to you to decide if it's worth it to hire a professional to negotiate debt settlement for you.

I highly recommend Dave Ramsey's programs and philosophy. I think he's got the right idea! Suze Orman also has great information in her books, and she has a television show. Jean Chatzsky's *Pay It Down! From Debt to Wealth in $10 a Day* has specific tools and strategies to help you as well. It's up to you to find someone whose tools, strategies and philosophy align with your own.

Avoiding Future Debt

"No." It's a complete sentence. It's your answer to, "Would you like to open a _____ charge account and save 10% today?" It's your answer to, "Would you like to use Visa or MasterCard today?" It's your answer to, "Should we eat out tonight?"

Unless, of course, you have a debit Visa or MasterCard, preferably one that provides cash back based on your usage, then go for it!

Get rid of all of your credit cards, save one. You should have one that's available to use when you travel. Hotels put a hold on more than the anticipated amount owed, which ties up your cash if you use a debit card, and can take days to "get back." It's good to purchase airline tickets and rent vehicles using a credit card as well. The rest of the time, use a debit card linked to your checking account, which means when you buy it, it's paid for. No big bill coming later for you to worry about. If you have it in your possession, it belongs to you and there's no worrying to be done.

Be sure you bank with a bank that protects you in the event your card is lost or stolen. I've had my card in my possession and someone has managed to get the number and buy some first-class airline tickets to Indonesia, but my bank protects it's members from this type of theft and fraud.

Clear Communication

It doesn't matter whom you owe money to, part of moving from debt into abundance is communicating where you are and what your plans are to pay your creditors back. There's nothing worse than no communication at all, especially to the person or company who is waiting for their money.

You've gotten into debt; now you get to own it and move forward. Part of moving forward is reaching out to your creditors and telling them what you can and will do.

Just after becoming a single mom, I was rushed to the hospital with, what turned out to be, a severe brain infection. Like many single moms, I ignored "not feeling well" until it turned into something that ultimately could have killed me (note: don't wait!). I had medical insurance that I had purchased for myself, but the insurance company refused to pay its portion and meaning I received a bill for $4,700. Well, at the time, I didn't have $4,700 unless I borrowed on credit, and I certainly didn't want to pay even more for the experience!

I knew for sure, no matter what, I could pay them $100 a month for 47 months. My intention was to pay them off sooner (and I did). After making my plan, I called their accounting department, told them I was a single mom and not only did I not expect to be sick, I also didn't expect my insurance company not to pay. I told them I would pay them every single month until the debt was satisfied, and sooner if I could. I also sent them something in writing and then scheduled a monthly payment through my online bill pay service. I did get a statement from them every month, but they never called me again.

A little known fact is that if you are making an effort to pay off your debts, your creditors aren't going to hammer you. It's when you avoid their calls, statements, and demand letters that they really get really update. Even if you can't pay right now, send them a letter and tell them so. Tell them what you're doing, explain your situation, and let them know you'll either (a) start making payments by a certain date or (b) send them an update in 60-90 days.

Just a Note

I'm not suggesting you eat only at home, never use credit, or do without every single luxury you can imagine. I'm just suggesting that if you have debt, there's a mental shift you should make if you want to get out of it and get out of it sooner. There may be deeper, psychological issues associated with your debt, and if you think that's true, find a therapist or coach to guide you through the process of changing what you believe about money and, effectively, what you believe about you and what you deserve.

In the Chapter 9, I'm going to share with you my abundance-creating results right away if you're open to giving them a try.

CHAPTER SIX

CREATING WEALTH:
YOU'VE GOT OPTIONS!

Now for the fun part: creating your riches! By now you've taken stock of where you are, figured out how you want your financial situation to be, and taken steps to move forward. What comes next is up to you, and you get to design it! Isn't that fantastic? You are the architect of your life and your future, and because we're specifically dealing with riches, wealth and abundance in this book, next we're going to explore your options.

I believe getting rich is done in stages, which starts right from where you are, seeing where you want to go next, and begin taking steps in that direction.

The Stages

Wherever you are, that's where you are and that is just fine! Accept it, focus on what you want next, and move forward.

Stage One: In debt. As previously discussed, while

starting to save you will be simultaneously paying any money you owe to anyone. Get your plan in place, communicate with your creditors, set up automatic payments, and then forget about them! Check in with what's happening once a month when you pay your bills, just so you can be aware of your progress.

Stage Two: At zero. Congratulations! You don't owe unsecured debt, and perhaps you have a little in reserve. Believe it or not, this is a dream for some people!

Stage Three: The Safety Net. Next, you want to keep saving until you have three to six months of living expenses in liquid cash. That means you can access it anytime you want without delay. Keep this money in a savings account. You won't yield much on your money, but you can get it when you need it.

Stage Four: Your War Chest. Once you have your Safety Net, then you can get into more advanced financial maneuvers. You'll want to do this with the help of your Dream Team, of course. The money in your War Chest is the money you're saving and investing that's in excess of your liquid capital. This is where your financial advisor comes into play, and where you'll be making long-term decisions about your retirement, including what you leave to your children. You won't touch this money for many years, so psychologically set yourself up with the belief that this isn't money you're going to use, no matter what. The exception to that is an opportunity to dip into your war chest to earn a significant return on an investment, or to help you overcome a major challenge. Be sure to have your Dream Team review these opportunities and listen to their advice. I have several formerly rich friends who thought they were financially bulletproof who are now rebuilding their wealth. That's no good, and certainty not fun!

The idea is to focus on what you want to do to eventually create your war chest. Do you have significant opportunities in your current job or business? Do you need a different job or career? Would you like to start your own business?

Some soul-searching might be in order here. Regardless of how you became a single mom, chances are there was a least some trauma or tragedy involved. You get the opportunity to reflect as well as take some time to look ahead into your future.

The Bill of Goods

In my work as an executive coach, I work with professionals who are already successful, some are even mega-successful, yet I have heard a common theme over the years about the bill of goods they've been sold about what they thought their lives would be like.

If I get a degree, a good job, make some money, get married, get a house, buy some cars, and have some kids, I'll be happy. However, after they check all those boxes, there is a feeling of discontent or downright unhappiness. We believe what we're told and when we don't feel the way we think we're supposed to feel, well then, now what?

Does this scenario sound familiar?

If so, you may need to hear you have the right to make any changes you deem necessary for your mental, physical, spiritual, and financial health. As I've said before, you get to make choices and decisions surrounding your future and what you want to do.

Said another way, if you feel stuck, you don't have to stay stuck. You aren't doomed to a life in a job that pays (or doesn't) well, miserably, and resentfully. If you want an education, you can go get one. (I'll explore your education options in a future book.) If you want to start your own business, you can do that, too.

Let's begin to explore your options, and before we do, meet Kristen Brown.

Successful Single Mom Kristen Brown's Story, Part I

Kristen Brown's single mom journey began unexpectedly when her husband died suddenly. A former college athlete, he was just thirty years old, leaving Kristen with an infant.

Kristen worked in corporate America and got an unsympathetic new boss just two weeks after her husband's death. This caused her stress level to skyrocket and to begin a period of introspection. The combination of the stress of her job and boss, the insurance company doing a complete investigation, and her own mourning process was the catalyst to her coming to the realization she needed to do something different. Kristen explains, "I didn't want my daughter to think back and think I was anything other than a role model. That launched me into what I'm doing today." She took a surf trip to Costa Rica with some girlfriends, and when she came home, she knew she had transformed into a different person.

"I started experimenting with stress management without really wanting to start a business. I had lost 20 pounds, and knew I needed to do something, but didn't want to go on anti-depressant or sleep aids. I started experimenting with meditation, yoga, exercise, vitamins, herbs and over-the-counter supplements to help me deal with the damage of stress. Within a year and a half, I realized there wasn't anything in the market that helps people holistically with stress. There are drugs and over-the-counter "Band-Aids" that come without the tools to help you be proactive when stress happens," shares Kristen.

What happened next changed her destiny, and serves as a model for anyone who wants to bring a new solution to the marketplace.

Since she didn't know exactly what to do next, she took small steps. Kristen went online and Googled "health supplements." Eventually, she had an FDA-approved lab help to formulate health supplement. At the exact same time, she was realizing her time in the corporate world had come to an end; her stress level was so high she knew it was a must to do something different. "The worst thing was I'd lose my home, all my money and live in my parents basement," she says. "The next day, I gave two weeks notice!"

Stay tuned, there's more of her story in an upcoming chapter.

CHAPTER SEVEN

CREATING WEALTH: WORK

Would it surprise you to learn that work is actually just one way of creating wealth and riches? There are other options, and we'll explore those, but this chapter is about your good old-fashioned do work-for-pay options.

I'm exploring these options because I want you to know what's available for you, as well as the up-sides and downsides of each option. There is no right or wrong answer here; it's just what's right or wrong for you.

Just like in everything else, what works for each individual is personal. Read and decide what resonates with you. Then, move forward when you are filled with all of the emotions that fill us up when we're embarking on a new journey: excitement, apprehension, enthusiasm, and passion.

Work for Someone Else

This is option one. Your current job or position is one

valid option for creating riches. Blooming where you're planted is a terrific idea. Taking it as far as it will take you can be energizing on a daily basis, fulfilling over the long-term, and financially fantastic for you.

Do you have a job you're thrilled about? Great! Your best bet then is to maximize your position, making yourself indispensible to your employer. In fact, do well enough and someday you might even own the company!

This section is understandably shorter than the upcoming section on being self-employed, mostly because of my passion for working for myself and encouraging others to do the same.

It needs to be noted; however, that as a single mom, you have many additional stressors and responsibilities, so solid, steady employment and the check that goes with it can be just the foundation you need in order to be a successful, **happy** single mom. Being successful and happy is not to be downplayed or diminished. It's truly important that you are happy, and I truly believe a happy mom perpetuates and allows for a happy kid. When I'm happy, I'm more patient, kind and tolerant than when I am not. I believe my daughter benefits directly, indirectly, implicitly, and explicitly because I'm happy.

Work for Yourself

I'm so excited about exploring this option with you! I've worked for major corporations, small businesses, and myself. By far, working for myself has been the most challenging, hardest, and one of the best things I have ever done. I enjoy the freedom, income, flexibility and most of all, time with my family.

To satisfy my pragmatic side, let's begin the analysis by dropping the gushy prose about the joys of self-realization that abound in working for yourself and about how "the real you" will bubble up from the depths when you control your own destiny. Instead I want to show you some of the considerations you need to face if you are thinking about going into business for yourself, and whether this option is the right step for you. There are a host of factors, personal and professional, in a decision about whether to go solo.

Some of them are:

- Situational: As a single mom, you have special family responsibilities. Do you have support from friends and family?

- Talents & Abilities: Do you have the skills to make it on your own?

- Psychological: Do you have the temperament and the discipline necessary to be successful?

- Financial: Do you have the money you need to get started? Or have enough saved to keep you afloat until your venture runs smoothly?

- Benefits: Are employee benefits available through your ex-spouse's employment (and are they in your Divorce Decree or Separation Agreement)? Can you afford to pay for health coverage, or can you take the risk of being without it?

- Legal: Do you understand and can you handle your increased liability as an independent professional? Can you afford to create the necessary legal documents (such as an LLC), and do you know the right person to help you?

• Ownership: Do you understand the differences as to who owns your work -- the copyright or patent or recipe -- if you create your creation as an employee? As a self-employed person? As a work-for-hire?

• The Unknown: How prepared are you for an emergency, such as being hurt while working? A long bout with the flu? A shortage of clients? Computer crashes? Car breakdowns? A no-show babysitter?

Whether to be self-employed or work for someone else: that's a choice that only you can make, one with no right or wrong answer.

Disadvantages of Self-Employment

All the important disadvantages of self-employment can be summed as one big piece of bad news: nobody is taking care of you. There's no "big daddy" to turn to, even if you can turn to your daddy. You alone are responsible for yourself – and often for a lot of others, too.

You are not paid for sick days; you must come up with the money to pay for your own health insurance; if you have a question about pensions you can't run to the personnel office on the 6th floor to get an answer; and there's no child-care subsidy. I am not saying that every employee has this kind of coverage and benefits, but I am saying that no one who is self-employed has them.

When you work for yourself you have no boss. You are both employer and employee, and in your dual role, you must pay both the employee's share and the employer's share of Social Security and Medicare tax, called Self-

Employment Tax.

As for your war chest, every penny comes from you, whereas in many companies employers contribute to the pensions and retirement accounts of their employees.

If you can't work or there is no work you don't get paid, and you can't apply for unemployment benefits, nor can you get Worker's Compensation for a work-related injury.

You are truly on your own.

It sounds daunting; but most intelligent independent professionals have faced all these considerations and have decided, as I did, that since we only live once, being your own boss is more fulfilling and more fun!

Advantages of Self-Employment

Now that we got the disadvantages out of the way, let's talk about the good stuff! The same things that make self-employment scary are also what make it attractive and adventurous. Nobody will take care of you, but instead of dwelling on that as bad news, embrace it as good news: it means you will be in charge, and in control of your destiny! Good stuff!

More good stuff: you will be responsible for yourself – and often for others, too. No big daddy, no anybody really, will tell you what to do, how to do it, and when to do it. Nor can anyone fire you. You'll have more control of your time and your life. I'm talking practicality here, not psychobabble about women running with the coyotes or adolescent rebelliousness and your contempt for "the suits."

Here's what I'm talking about. Do you want to work until three in the morning all week so that you can take four days off to go skiing? You can. Do you want to start the day late so you can have breakfast with your children? You can. Do you want to do a reassessment, realignment, and redirect of your focus and direction? You can! If you're not feeling great and want to work from your home in your PJ's, you can. You can fit your schedule into the schedule of the kids, maybe eliminating the need for expensive or inadequate childcare. If you have a great idea, you can try it. If it doesn't work, you are responsible for that too, but you can make changes and improve your idea without the need to play company politics with the sales department down the hall.

Also with self-employment comes financial advantages. One of the less obvious advantages is the possibility of more money for the same work. Many companies have downsized (don't you love that word?) and former employees have been fired, and then engaged as independent contractors. Why do you think that has happened? Money! It saves the company a big bundle – in payroll taxes and benefits – to hire someone as a freelancer rather than as an employee. Should you work for the same fee that you would be paid as an employee? No, you shouldn't. You should ask for more. You are costing them less than a full-time employee, how about splitting the difference? If you're engaged by someone who has never run a business or never hired anyone to work for him, maybe you'll need to point out the financial savings to him and why he should use your services instead of those of the temp agency he's considering.

Self-employment comes with tax advantages as well. You are in control, so in many instances …

- You have more influence over business expense deductions.

- More business expenses are actually deductible.

- You get more flexibility in how much tax you'll

pay and when you'll pay it.

• You get to decide when to spend money to help your business grow.

• You can influence when you receive income.

• You can distribute income to family members by hiring them as employees.

• You have a wide range of pension choices.

There are many options for self-employment and we're going to discuss a few of them here. Once you read about something that intrigues you or gets you excited, do your due diligence and then take whatever steps you can to move forward. Think hard about it, but don't think too long. The most successful people make decisions quickly and are slow to change them. They stick to their guns and allow for no Plan B. When you're ready to do that, you're ready.

Success Starts with Attitude

I would be remiss if I didn't put work and your attitude about work into perspective and share some professional insights with you.

The clients I have that own their companies love nothing more than employees who take ownership and stewardship over their positions. These are the employees who act as if they own the company, meaning that they show up on time or early, have a can-do attitude all day, every day, spend the company's resources as if the money was coming out their own pocket, and do more than they are paid to do. There is always room for advancement for the person who is willing to contribute more than what's expected.

It's kind of like when your kids do something without you having to ask, or they do a little something extra. After you've picked yourself up off the floor, aren't you really proud? Don't you want to do a little something special for them? Aren't you so excited and thrilled? I know I am.

"He Who Never Does More Than He Gets Paid For, Never Gets Paid For More Than He Does!"

The problem I see sometimes in the people I'm hired to coach is that they don't have a can-do attitude. They want all of the features and benefits of being the boss, they want to make more money today but they haven't paid their dues. What they don't know or see in its entirety is how hard the boss has had to work over a span of years (yes, years) and works to make it all happen (and probably make their job look easy).

Now, if you have a bad boss who wears cranky pants every single day, hardly works at all, and makes millions of dollars, all I can say is he is the exception, not the rule. I advise you to find another job immediately in which you can excel.

The truth is if you are the cranky person, you need to be elsewhere. Staying at a job you don't enjoy in the slightest is a disservice to yourself and your boss. If you can't or won't show up and do the job you were paid to do, go somewhere else. If you can't give a little extra because you can and, in my opinion, you should, then you need to be actively seeking other employment. If you are using company time and resources to do anything other than your job (Facebooking, personal phone calls, smoke breaks, extra long lunches, etc.), you are stealing from your employer and the company, and you need to go! You deserve better, and this behavior isn't indicative of someone who is happy and in the right place. Your employer deserves better, too: he deserves to get what he is paying to get.

As a side note, it's impossible to be your best when you are around toxic people and if you have a toxic boss, it is virtually impossible to excel.

The cream always rises to the top, and doing your job and more will assure that (a) you have a job, (b) your boss(es) will appreciate you and reward you at their every opportunity, and (c) you will have the cash you need ultimately to create the wealth picture you painted for yourself in an earlier chapter.

As a self-employed single mom, you'll need to take the above-mentioned super qualities for an employee and magnify them to succeed in your own gig.

To work for yourself, you've got to feel unstoppable, have a reserve of can-do attitude and generous helpings of passion and purpose. Because you're human and humans all have "bad days," you'll have one, too, from time to time.

Let me let you in on a little secret. Whether someone else currently employs you, or your name is on the door, you are working for yourself. You are in essence YOU, Inc., and your success, while affected by others, is ultimately up to you. You need to, if you don't have them already, nurture and expand those positive qualities, no matter who signs your paycheck.

Working For Yourself: The Benefits

As a single mom, being self-employed is in many ways, the perfect marriage. Pun intended. When you work for yourself, you have control over what probably stresses you out the most as a single mom: time and money.

As a self-employed person, you can potentially and will most-likely make more money than being employed. While it's true that you 'eat what you kill,' meaning that you make it, so you get to control the majority of it, and more often than not those profits end up in your own wallet.

Most of the time, you can mold your schedule around your children's schedules. I have missed very few of Lexi's activities, and I've been able to attend every parent-teacher conference, concert, play performance, belt test, holiday party, graduation, and field trip. That is a pretty cool feeling, and I know she's been excited to have me there every time.

Here's the disclaimer: self-employment is not for the faint of heart. You have never worked harder in your life! But if you're willing to combine your passion with the commitment to success, and you seek out good guidance and advice, you can't help but be successful.

Single Mom Cassie Boorn's Story

Cassie Boorn is a 23-year-old single mom, who, in her short years, has already figured out a way to support her son (Aiden, now age 5) while working in her PJ's, and living in a small town.

In college, she worked at Pizza Hut, but she fostered dreams of supporting her son while working from home. She has admirably done exactly that: a graduate of St. Ambrose University, she is now the social media coordinator at DeVries Public Relations, and how she went from college student with dreams to employed on her terms provides many lessons for all of us.

Cassie said, "I wanted to work from home, and had started blogging. I discovered all these amazing women working from home, writing stories, and I wanted to be a part of it."

She reached out to bloggers, and during her searching process, found a woman putting on a conference and called her. She ended up being hired as the director of marketing for the site. In the midst of all of this, she started a project and asked women to write letters to their 20 something self, which was featured in the New York Times, had her interviewed on NPR and even securing a book deal!

"Still working at the restaurant, I was working on the side selling sponsorships and brands. It felt like I was doing something bigger and that felt empowering. I had dipped my toe into a new space and was acquiring new skills," she shared.

Cassie's words are filled with encouragement for single moms, "With the Internet and social media, you can start your own business, sell something like Avon or anything else you'd like. You have many channels, many options of working from home, in a small town, even with a company in a big city. The options are really there. Figuring out what you LOVE, if you LOVE music, food, or fashion, you can build anything around that and turn it into a career. It can be a side career at first, there's no need to quit your job, run through your savings, but build it slowly and then turn it into something without the risks you have as a single mom. There are options there, which is really cool."

Working For Yourself: The Options

There is a plethora of options when looking to start your own business. I have deep knowledge of two, and fairly good knowledge of the others. Here they are:

- Franchises

- Networking Marketing/Direct Sales

- Your own idea [inventions]

- Products

- Services

- Other options

Franchises

I borrowed this from the website Franchise Opportunities:

> *When selecting a franchise, carefully consider a number of factors, such as the demand for the products or services, likely competition, the franchisor's background, and the level of support you will receive. You also need to carefully consider how much money and time you are willing to invest in the franchise opportunity.*

To these words of wisdom, I will add: can you secure a great location, one that ensures high traffic. Also, I see Subway doing lots of promotion (on shows like my favorite The Biggest Loser); please consider what the franchisor will be doing to help your location as well.

You can select a franchise from $2,000 to over $1,000,000, but most franchises I looked into were between $20,000-$100,000. If you've found yourself as a single mom with capital, franchising might be an option for you. I personally know several individuals who have accumulated wealth by starting with one franchise and then adding to their "collection" of franchises over a period of years. One family I know even created a new franchise and became the franchisor! In both cases, once the right management team is in place, the business can run itself with very little owner input or involvement. You can choose to stay involved in the day-to-day of the business, or delegate running your business to a carefully selected team.

Network Marketing (a.k.a. MLM)

My personal experience in self-employment started at age 23 when I started my own network marketing business, with the Shaklee Corporation. My parents were educated professionals and entrepreneurs and their business of choice was network marketing, specifically with Shaklee. I feel like I chose the best, but this is certainly not a commercial for Shaklee. I'm sharing with you my experience, from my perspective, because that's all I can do. When making your decision, be sure to speak to as many people as you need to before you make your final decision. I no longer actively build a Shaklee business, but I still use and love the products and couldn't imagine using anything else. If you're interested specifically in Shaklee, please visit the Resources section for more information.

Network Marketing consists of companies that have a marketing strategy in which the sales force is compensated not only for sales they personally generate, but also for the sales of others they recruit, creating a downline of distributors and a hierarchy of multiple levels of compensation. Some of the top leaders in the industry are Shaklee, Mary Kay, NuSkin, and Avon.

When selecting a network marketing company, there are several factors that are important. If I were looking to build a new company from scratch today, I would recommend to you the same things I recommended to people looking at building a Shaklee business ten years ago. Look for a company with:

- An excellent reputation in Direct Sales, with the Better Business Bureau, and "on the street."

- The companies need a good, solid track record, preferably they've been in business for ten years or more

- The company should be 100% debt free

- Their compensation plan should be attainable and provide an equal opportunity for all distributors

- The best products to sell are consumable, meaning that your customers will need to buy them again, and repeat business is part of the power of Network Marketing.

- The products need to be safe for consumer, and better than the conventional products they can buy at the grocery store or at Target.

The Corporate Office should have a powerful team consisting of strong leadership. When the company decides to introduce new products or make a change in the compensation plan from time to time, you need to have full faith in their ability to make those decisions. This is because they affect you and your downline!

Interview your Upline. Ask to see a copy of their Bonus or Income Statements. The person who sponsors you doesn't need to be making a ton of money. He could be new and newly pursuing his dream team (you), but the Upline makes a huge difference about how seriously your prospects will take you and your opportunity. Choose someone you feel you can work well with because at least at first, you'll be spending quite a bit of time on the phone and doing meetings with him.

The company should have available affordable (or free) training and on-going support, business training, and product information. If you want information, you should have information. There should also be lots of training options: one-on-one training, group training, online training, and phone training. If you're an information person and you need and desire a lot of information, it needs to be easily accessible to you.

Both the business opportunity and the products should appeal to both sexes. In my opinion, make-up companies are fine and can check the rest of the boxes, but you've cut your possible demographic in half. A sound business decision for you could be to choose a company that appeals to everyone.

The company should provide excellent corporate support, hold the majority of the inventory, and do the lion's share of the product distribution. Your sole focus is sharing the business opportunity and sharing the products with possible consumers. They should be able to order the products online or over the phone and then shipped right to their door.

Finally, starting your business shouldn't cost a fortune! With any business, you should be willing and able to commit a fair sum (less than $1,000, in most cases around $500) to launch your business. It should be easy and affordable for you to begin.

Your Own Idea: A Life-Changing Invention

Moms are notorious (in a good way) for inventing really cool stuff. Remember Baby Einstein? I bought all of those videos for my daughter, and I have heard that millions of other moms did, too.

A product is really just a solution to a common problem. I read an interview with a mom inventor and she said, "All I had to do was pay attention when I had a problem, think about it, and try to solve it." You can do the same!

Because I haven't invented anything yet, I can only direct you to some amazing websites I found with a ton of information. Check the Resources Section for my recommendations.

Deciding to start a business is one thing. It's helpful to know that you might experience some unsettling emotions. Here's more about single mom Kristen Brown:

Successful Single Mom Kristen Brown's Story, Part II

"My first day of working for myself, I woke up, turned on computer and now what?" shares Kristen. "I had a mini freak out, thinking I'm starting my own deal. I wasn't an idiot, so I knew what I needed to be doing, but I'm my own person, I don't have to go to meetings, report to anyone."

She set up recurring weekly meeting with herself to review goals, look at her progress, and look at her to-do list. "I needed something to start with. Oprah said, 'schedule in me time' setting up meetings with herself for herself."

Kristen set up speaking engagements to talk about her story, which led to her releasing her book, The Happy Hour Effect in May 2011. Her mission is to help people realize stress is a big deal, it causes health problems, and there are healthy, practical solutions.

Products & Services: The Options are Limitless

You can retain your self-employed status while working under the structure of well-known companies with an independent sales force. New York Life and Colonial Life are two examples of insurance companies where you work for yourself but you have the solid reputation of an established, distinguished brand behind you. Truly, the only limits to the opportunities are the ones you impose on yourself. If you're sincerely open to working for yourself, begin to explore all of the options and when you find the one that will work for you, you'll know it. You can sell baskets from Longaberger Baskets, candles from Party Lite, and kitchen equipment from The Pampered Chef. There are branded and private-label personal products sold through Fuller Brush and vacuum cleaners for sale through Electrolux. I also found medical billing opportunities for single moms online, so do a search for different ideas, and you're sure to find something that might be a good fit.

Another option for you is to go into business for yourself providing a service, such as bookkeeping, house cleaning, or consulting. If you have an area of expertise you can generally find individuals and companies that are interested in what you have to offer and they certainly don't need a full-time person to do the job.

The trick is, I think, to translate something you love into what you get paid to do. I attended a Tony Robbins seminar in 1995 and I'll never forget a woman standing up and saying she absolutely loved to clean house. Her house, your house, my house, and she didn't mind cleaning it. Amazing! I'll do just about anything to get out of cleaning, but she loved it and said it literally made her happier than almost anything else she did. Go figure! She had a house-cleaning business that generated over a million dollars a year because not only did she clean, she found other people who loved to clean, too, and they created a magical synergy that led to clean homes for her clients and a giant bank account for her.

As for me, almost thirteen years ago, I reached a personal and professional turning point. I was given a coach by Shaklee and very soon reached my long-term goals in a much shorter period of time (about 90 days). The turning point caused deep reflection and an evaluation about how I wanted to spend my life, and what legacy I wanted to leave. My coach helped me to discover a love for coaching, speaking and training. She encouraged me to launch my own business, and with her guidance and support and many hours of immersion, I did. I shifted focus from my Shaklee business to actually coaching some of my customers. All these years later, I still can't wait to get out of bed each day and be a force for good. I can coach for seven hours straight with barely enough time to run to the bathroom in between sessions, throw down a protein shake for lunch, and end up more energized at the end of the day. Now, I can't vouch for my brain working all that well, but I'm raring to go, nonetheless. No day is the same, and thankfully, I get amazingly positive feedback about my work.

If there's something you absolutely love to do and if the thought of getting paid for it makes you giddy, then that is the thing you probably need to look into translating into your income.

Just think about a skill-set you've picked up along the way and get creative using the goal-setting process in Chapter 1 to release the ideas of your inner entrepreneur.

Before you poo-poo what it is you love to do, remember that people are paid for shopping and even for sleeping (think: sleep studies). Several years ago, I met a gal who provides "security" for warehouses. Once a week, for each property, she goes to the site, checks to make sure the locks are working, nothing has been disturbed and the dogs are still alive and kicking (someone else is in charge of feeding the dogs). The alarm company is set to call her if an alarm is tripped, but says it's only happened four times in three years. She's got enough clients that she supports herself and her two small children. Talk about freedom and flexibility! She only works a few hours a week and is free to be a great mom the rest of the time to her kids.

Successful Single Mom Julie Pech's Story

Julie Pech is the author of a book called The Chocolate Therapist: A User's Guide to the Extraordinary Health Benefits of Chocolate. She speaks up to twenty times a month about the benefits of chocolate, teaches about chocolate and wine, and chocolate and tea pairings. She also hosts corporate and charity events and travels as a guest lecturer on cruise ships teaching classes about chocolate. She also own a chocolate shop where she makes handcrafted, all-natural chocolate candies with nuts, berries, spices and organic flavoring oils to support the concepts in her book. She's been a single mother for six years, and her kids are now 14 and 16. Julie says, "They have seen me go through everything!"

Julie shares her experience: "I left my very unhealthy marriage right in the middle of writing my book. I had no income, and I really had to make a leap of faith that I was on the right track. Everyone told me to get a real job and stop chasing dreams, but I couldn't do it. I had the blinders on and I was going forward!

"I wrote the book, started speaking to get the word out, launched a little chocolate line to go with the book, and then ended up buying the shop that was making my line. There was so much serendipity that I couldn't possibly have planned. I believe this happens whenever someone has the courage to embrace what she is truly called to do. Being heart-driven brings extraordinary luck. When I speak to women's groups, I say, "Your herd is out there waiting for you, they're just on the other side of the hill. You can't see them until you're moving forward. Go for your dreams and the people you need will come into your life."

"For example, after working extremely hard for 4 years, I'd sold 6,000 copies of my self-published book. I decided it was time to find a real publisher, but I wanted to go on a horseback-riding retreat in Wyoming for a week as kind of a self-gift. I committed to finding a publisher on my return, and as it turned out, I met the publisher on my trip!"

Julie always knew she wanted to be a writer and had launched that plan when her marriage was falling apart. Now, as a single mom, she's living into that vision. She keeps her monthly nut small, which she knows is a long-term play. She's working toward creating something huge that she can sell later. As she told me, "You live lean in the beginning, but still give yourself small rewards along the way. Later when the payoff comes, treat yourself to something wonderful." Her affordable reward: extraordinary chocolate, of course!

Julie's self-care is inspiring: She takes Fridays off. She recommends you choose a day and make it about you. It will change your life. She gets up early and focuses on honoring her own needs throughout the day. "I didn't realize how valuable it was to have a full day to myself until I tried it. But even if you can only spare half a day, do it. Choose something that's not too expensive that you love to do. Get a massage, have your nails done, go on an intense bike ride, it's worth every minute. I know I'm a better mother now because I spend time loving myself. I've only been doing it for a year and I'm more relaxed and focused, which helped improve my relationship with my kids as well." Thanks for that tidbit of wisdom, Julie!

What's next? Julie's writing a book about embracing turning fifty. Aging gracefully without going broke, you don't really need Botox, liposuction, and so forth. It's about beautiful aging with just diet, exercise, and hydration and how your life can get better instead of worse as you age instead of worse. I, for one, can't wait to get my hands on that book!

Business Plan

It's crucial to have a well thought-out, written business plan before you launch a business. Your written plan describes your business, outlines your goals, and serves as a road map for future activities, including everything from handling unforeseen complications to repaying borrowed money. It is a document that can and will grow with your business, undergoing constant tweaks and revisions as your big idea evolves from a concept into a successful company.

A strong business plan is essentially the cornerstone of your business, but many budding business owners drag their feet when it comes to writing one, possibly because it involves a good deal of work and may bring back childhood memories of writing a tedious book report on summer vacation. It is critical that you not only organize your thoughts on how you intend to run your business but also formalize your plan in writing. Here's why:

- **A business plan forces you to identify your and your company's strengths and weaknesses.** You don't want to start a company that is flawed before it is even in business. Sitting down, writing a plan, thinking about everything you bring to the table (whether that's a passion for cupcakes or an enthusiasm for medical software) and considering everything you're lacking (whether that's salesmanship or computer skills) can give you a realistic snapshot of your odds of success. Your goal should be to focus on your strengths and fix any problems that could hamper your growth.

- **A business plan helps you figure out how much money you will need.** Entrepreneurs chronically underestimate how much money they'll need to start a business. Keep in mind that a lack of capital is one of the top reasons why businesses struggle or close during the first year. Writing a plan forces you to get a handle on where your money will come from, where it will go, and whether it will be enough, not only to get your business off the ground, but also to sustain growth in subsequent years. As a single mom, there are significant, special resources available to you to help you attain this money.

• **A business plan gives you clear direction, which can help alleviate or eliminate stress.** As a business owner, you often initially juggle multiple roles -- everything from bookkeeper to CEO -- and those roles can leave you feeling distracted, disorganized, and overwhelmed. A document that outlines your mission and plans for the future can help prevent overload, set realistic goals, keep you on track, and significantly boost your productivity.

• **A business plan will serve as a resume when you seek lenders, investors or partners.** Most lenders, and certainly any professional investor, such as an angel or venture capitalist, will expect to see a business plan before giving you money. Even if you are not seeking outside money, a business plan can be helpful when renting space (a landlord might ask to see one) or seeking a business partner. For partners who start a business together, writing a plan ensures that everyone is on the same page when it comes to the company's mission, everyone's roles, the big goals, strategies and tactics.

- **A business plan makes you evaluate the market for your product or service and size up the competition.** As you write your plan, you will research the current market and see how your product or service might fare against existing offerings. By analyzing your competition, you will get a sense of how to price your product or service, how to target the right customers, and how to make your company stand out, particularly in a crowded marketplace. As you assemble your business plan, you will see opportunities to fine-tune your concept, avoid problems that could become disasters, and ultimately increase your odds of success.

Action Plan

Once you have completed your Business Plan, I advise you to create an Action Plan for your next step. I personally work in 100-day increments, and that's also how I work with my coaching clients. I chose 100 days for a few reasons, and here's the main one: I hate math. For each goal, you track where you are percentage-wise on a daily basis. If want to make $100,000 in 100 days, that's $1,000 per day. On day 36, I should have made $36,000. If I've made $30,000, I'm 6% behind, at $50,000, I'm 14% ahead. Simple, right? It's always best to keep it simple. Reason number two, 100 days is long enough to accomplish something, but not too long that you lose focus. I think New Year's Resolutions are terrific, but I only think about them on New Year's. There's no "check in on how my resolutions are going" on a regular basis. No reviewing what you're after is one reason they don't work for most people.

In your Business Plan, the focus is what happens overall,

long-term in your business. Your Action Plan is what you're going to do to bring that vision to fruition, over a shorter period of time.

You can download a free copy of my 100-Day Action Plan from my website at http://www.coachhonoree.com/resources.

Financing for Single moms

A good bet for you to raise capital for your business might be an SBA guaranteed loan for as much as $750,000 for a term of seven years. Call the SBA field office nearest you or call the SBA Answer Desk at 800.368.5855. Two good general pamphlets describing SBA loan functions are "Business Loans from the SBA" and "Your Business and the SBA."

You can also find financing through private investors, angel groups or even other successful entrepreneurs!

CHAPTER EIGHT

CREATING WEALTH: HABITS

If there's one thing Andrew Carnegie had, it was a set of unwavering beliefs. Regardless of what obstacles stood in his way, his characteristics and habits allowed him to overcome all of them. It was his belief in himself and his abilities that allowed him to go from a worker in a bobbin factory to a Captain of Industry in the steel industry. Andrew Carnegie's life is a testament of a true "rags to riches" story. Like most rich and wealthy individuals, Carnegie spent his life developing characteristics and habits that allowed him to become one of the most powerful, influential and wealthiest individuals of his time. The only thing that separated him from everyone else, including you, was his beliefs.

Understand that the characteristics and habits of the rich and wealthy are defined by their beliefs. Your beliefs and habits will define your wealth.

It's possible for you to have everything Carnegie had, and more, as long as you adopt the characteristics and habits of the rich and wealthy. But most importantly, you must believe that you deserve to achieve your dreams and goals.

You see, people of poverty, strain and struggle to hold a state of mind of lack and scarcity. They don't believe there is an abundance of love, success, money, happiness, and everything else they desire in life, but there is.

On the other hand, the rich and wealthy hold a state of mind of prosperity and abundance. They believe there is an infinite source that provides them with everything they desire. They don't allow themselves ever to think that there will never be enough of what they need to be successful.

So it goes without saying that if you hold a certain set of beliefs, then you will exhibit certain characteristics and habits.

Below are eight of the most common characteristics and habits extremely rich people have, beliefs that you will need to adopt if you truly desire to be rich and wealthy:

1. Making money is extremely easy, and money comes easily and frequently.

2. Keeping and growing my money is extremely easy.

3. There's an abundance of money and resources.

4. I'm a financial genius.

5. When I focus on a goal, it's as good as done.

6. Failure is a learning lesson.

7. I can do anything.

8. I'm incredibly self-disciplined.

Another characteristic the rich and wealthy have is

the ability to understand how to leverage their efforts for the most gain in the shortest possible period of time. Their understanding of leverage that allows the money to pour in by the boatloads.

While adopting these beliefs is doable, you must commit a considerable amount of effort into altering the deep-rooted subconscious beliefs you currently have about success and money.

If you continue to allow the irrational beliefs of your childhood to guide you throughout life, then life will appear to be hard. In my humble opinion, that's the way you want it because easy come, easy go. You will (continue to) hinder yourself from receiving the type of lifestyle you desire and undoubtedly deserve. Or, you can identify those limiting beliefs, see them for the nonsense they are, and decide to adopt some new beliefs. Just the eight beliefs above can and will make a positive difference for you. If you truly take on those beliefs, imagine how great life will be. Close your eyes, just for a moment, and picture what life is like when you believe, "I'm a financial genius and money is always coming to me easily and effortlessly." Sure a heck of a lot better than, "I hope I have enough to pay the rent this month."

Although I have never met you, I'm confident you can do whatever you set your mind to, but you must own your goals and dreams, and take personal responsibility to make them happen.

Success is possible! Remember this, it's easy to be a success. The hardest part is believing abundance, success, and wealth can happen for you.

Habits to Adopt ASAP

1. Start early: First things first, start your kids out

early on the road to sound financial management. When you equip your kids with the right attitude and habits about money, you'll leave them with lifelong financial lessons that help them develop a strong sense of self-reliance. Jeff Bogle of Stop Buying Crap suggests one way for parents is to be able to integrate financial lessons with children's playtime.

2.   Take tips from weight loss: Just as we should work to educate our children on money, we should continue developing our own money-management skills. To improve ourselves in general, especially in our fiscal discipline, take a lesson from those who lose weight over time: they assign a measure to what they want, they take action daily, and they check in regularly.

3.   Get things for less: On that note, there's another set of skills that may serve you well as a consumer. By learning how to negotiate, haggle, or barter, you can stretch your budget much farther. This kind of resourcefulness has allowed many a family to live below their means while still being able to enjoy great deals, creature comforts and a self sustaining lifestyle.

4.   Earn a bit extra: Open your mind to additional streams of income. As discussed in the previous chapter, you can take a passion, interest, or hobby and develop it into a money making channel.

5.   Get rich, slowly: Most people think they could never make $1 million in their life, let alone in

a year's time. They believe becoming wealthy is something that's just way too hard to do. At the same time, we want to gravitate towards the path of least resistance. No surprise that "get rich quick schemes" (such as the lottery or slot machines) are so popular. Many fall prey to scams or hope to inherit a windfall, all in the pursuit of the quick buck. You would do better to create your plan and then consistently and ruthlessly work that plan. Make money, buy what you need and want within reason, save a percentage of your income, and use your Dream Team to multiply what you have.

6.   Hang out with your rich friends, or, make some new rich friends. Speaking of getting rich, your income tends to be right about the same as the people you hang out with the most. My dear friend Scott said one of his secrets of wealth is to hang out consistently with people who make $100,000 a month, month in and month out. What do you think they discuss? How they are making, giving, saving, and investing their money, of course. What do the strugglers discuss? Why they have so little money and those damn rich people have so much! Do surround yourself with such abundant friends, if you have them. Their "wealth mentality" could very well, and will most likely, rub off on you. It never hurts to surround yourself with people who inspire you to action. This will help you to believe in yourself, and know what you want is possible.

7.   Learn to read your bank, investment and

financial statements. Initially, stash your savings from your extra income into a low cost bank account that pays a good interest rate. Although it's not something many of us do religiously, it's still a wise idea to learn how to read our bank statements. Pay attention to each fee and if you can, bank with a bank that pays you back ATM fees and offers a percent back to you of what you spend each month.

8.   Your "babies need to be making babies." No, not your actual babies! The money you make, those first pennies, nickels and dimes you put away will eventually multiply over time through the beautiful concept called compound interest. The more you can put away, the more those dollars and cents will be working for you, no matter what you're doing.

The message here is to keep learning and keep doing. Even if you didn't get a chance to start early, it's never too late to build a foundation in personal finance through the habits you develop. What's important is to start somewhere, to make a decision to take your finances seriously, and to stay dedicated to your goals. Consistency is key!

Successful Single Mom Nancy D. Butler's Story

Nancy Butler's single mom story began in 1981, when her daughters were 8 and 15. Working in the same industry as her husband and in the process of a divorce, Nancy knew she had to change everything about her life, and discover who she was and what she liked.

She had allowed her husband to control every aspect of her life, including what she wore, and how she styled her hair. She wore what he liked, and did what he wanted to do, therefore it was a liberating day when she discovered she was no longer accountable to him. She would finally get to decide what she wanted, how she wanted to do it, and when she would have it!

While in the process of divorce, Nancy took her 2 daughters and with no child support, alimony or other source of income, moved 70 miles away and started her own business. At the new location, she was offered a salaried position at a higher pay then she had ever had before, but realized they were hiring her at "the top of the ladder," leaving her no place to grow.

She did not want a job she needed a career! "I knew nothing about saving, investing or financial planning, and had never owned a CD, mutual fund or anything other than a savings account. I told myself that even if the business didn't work out, the knowledge and experience I would gain would be worth it since what I would learn about managing money would help me to raise my children," said Nancy. "I found that I really enjoyed helping others determine the goals that are most important to them and help them put a plan in place to accomplish those goals and be financially secure. I built the business from scratch to become one of the top asset management and financial planning practices in the country within the company. With approximately $200 million in assets under management and 1,200 clients, in 2007 I sold my practice."

Her life looks different today: since selling her company, she's enjoying the fruits of her labor. She has accumulated enough wealth that she doesn't have to work ever again if she doesn't want to, and she now provides inspiration around the country: "I am now a national speaker to help business owners do a better job for their clients and improve their bottom line. I help individuals live a successful life and realize their dreams. I remain one of the few Certified

Divorce Financial Analysts in my state." Nancy commented.

CHAPTER NINE

CREATING WEALTH:
MIND OVER MANIFESTING
(OR HAVING A MILLIONAIRE MINDSET)

While work and what you do play a part in your financial status, being rich ultimately comes down to your psychology. What you believe and how you feel greatly influence your financial success and abundance. You have in your life exactly what you believe you deserve. If you don't, right now, have everything you want, worry not! You can expand your thinking and expand your riches.

The best news ever is that success is an "inside job" and is determined more by what's between your ears and inside your heart than by what's outside of them.

The timeless classic, *Think and Grow Rich* by Napoleon Hill is a book I've read almost monthly since 1991. Every time I read it, I see something I "haven't seen before." I've benefited so much from that book and its predecessor, *Law of Success*, also by Napoleon Hill. You'll find both included in the Suggested Reading section.

The great Jim Rohn, father of personal development, once slightly changed Mr. Hill's recommendation to, "*Think* and you *will* be rich."

You Can Have What You Want

Catherine Ponder, my heroine of prosperous thinking, says, "You are prosperous to the degree that you are experiencing peace, health, and plenty in your world."

A law is a principle that works, a settled rule of action. A law suggests desire for order, and it's non-negotiable. There are the laws that we live by daily, such as scientific laws, traffic laws, and criminal laws. Let's go even further. There are also higher mental and spiritual laws than those usually used on the physical plane of life. These higher mental and spiritual laws are so powerful that they can be used to multiply, neutralize, or even reverse natural laws! When we use these higher mental and spiritual laws they often produce results that seem miraculous on the physical plane.

To begin to change your beliefs about riches, wealth, and money, you must establish a definite pattern of prosperous thinking. In other words, you must be absolutely conscious of your thoughts and create daily thought habits to keep you on the right track. In essence and in reality, your thoughts determine what happens next. Isn't it true that you thought about getting this book, and then you got it? You thought about what you were going to eat for breakfast, and then you ate it. Our thoughts precede everything that happens. Make the connection between your thoughts and your beliefs, and between your beliefs and your outcomes. When you do, you can intentionally choose your thoughts, beliefs and outcomes. I don't know about you, but when I really grasped that concept, it was a true a-ha moment for me. I was thrilled that no matter what had already happened, I had a say in what was going to happen.

But how?

I have more great news for you: the how is not hard. The how is simple and easy, and it can be done in just minutes a day. What's the trick? I promise, there is no trick. You simply must dedicate some mental time every day to creating your riches. You must dedicate some time to feeling physically great. Combine the two and you will feel unstoppable, especially if the situation you're in is particularly challenging right now and you don't see any way out of it.

Additionally, you're going to go about your business and continue working in your job or business.

While I love the Law of Attraction, I don't believe you sit and think about money and it falls from the sky. I do believe that I can sit and think good thoughts about money, and then after I've become clear about how much I want, need, and would like to have, I've got to get moving and shake my money maker! I believe I've got to take action, get moving, and take the first of many steps. Thinking right and acting right is the power couple of success, a truly magical combination.

Seriously, everything you want will come easier when you think right, but you've also got to act right, too.

> *"Vision without action is merely a dream.*
> *Action without vision just passes the time.*
> *Vision with action can change the world."*
> ~Joel Barker

Why?

Why not? Why wouldn't you try what others have tried and swear by? I hear almost daily from single moms who are looking for the spring in their step. They used to have a joy for life that's disappeared, and they want it back! When you begin to put your new prosperity skills into action, you will have a new look, which comes from inner peace, poise, happiness, security, and stability.

The Outrageous Truth About Wealth and You

The shocking truth about wealth is that it is shockingly right, instead of shockingly wrong for you to be prosperous.

In his **Acres of Diamonds** lecture, Russell H. Conwell said:

> *"I say you ought to be rich; you have no right to be poor. To live and not be rich is a misfortune and it is doubly a misfortune because you could have been rich just as well as being poor. We ought to get rich if we can by honorable methods, and these are the only methods that sweep us quickly toward the goal of riches."*

You should desire riches, wealth, and abundance. It is your right to be rich! Rich means an abundance of good, or living a fuller, more satisfying life.

Wouldn't you agree that lack of money causes many of the social challenges, which result from fear and lack (crime, drugs, alcohol abuse, suicide, etc.)? You yourself may feel uncomfortable, stressed, and degraded, but those feelings are insane!

I truly believe you cannot live fully without being rich. You can't contribute to others if you're barely making ends meet. *You do not have to buy into the fact that because you're a single mom, you're doomed to a life of struggle.*

On the Physical Plane, you need and deserve food, clothing and shelter. On the Mental Plane, you need and deserve books, music, art, travel, intellectual associations, friendships, deep meaningful relationships, and so forth. On the Spiritual Plan, you need and deserve quiet contemplation, prayer, church, and meditation.

In other words, you are unable to contribute fully to yourself and others all of the things you want to have, do, be and create in the world if you live in lack. Life is too short to live in lack! You can do so much more for yourself and your kids when you live in abundance and it's your right to be abundant!

Make no further excuses to yourself and others for wanting to be prosperous. Whatever you believe, recognize that God or the Universe is the source of your supply and that there is always a supply for every demand. If you're not religious or don't believe in God, substitute whatever word is comfortable to you.

If you want it, you can have it!

There's a rich supply is all around you universally, as well as innately within you, such as talents, abilities, and ideas longing for expression, however that rich supply and substance must be contacted and used. Your mind is your connecting link with them. Your attitudes, your mental concepts, beliefs, and outlook are your connecting links to this rich substance and are your access to it. Prosperous and abundant thinking opens the way to prosperous results.

Coach's Note: Don't be surprised when you start to get some really cool and unexpected results almost right away.

The Basic Law of Wealth

The power of our thinking is an instrument for success or failure. As I've said before, at the very least, first and foremost, you must gain control of your thoughts and get those thoughts thinking about what you truly want.

Remember I said this process was simple and easy? How's this for simple: beginning to become more prosperous is as easy as deciding you wish to be more prosperous. Your potential health, wealth and happiness are within you, waiting to be radiated to the outside world thereby attracting what you desire. That decision can take you less than a second, so whenever you're ready, go ahead, I'll wait.

The basic law of wealth is "radiation" and "attraction." You've heard it as sowing and reaping, giving and receiving, or supply and demand. Emerson referred to it as the Law of Compensation: like attracts like.

Whatever you radiate outward in your thoughts, feelings, mental pictures, and words, you attract into your life. To activate this radiation, there is always something you can do to begin the process. I recommend you start with daily actions, like the ones I'll share shortly.

Here's the truth: you are already using radiation and attraction because you are a magnet. The question is, what are you a magnet for? What are you currently attracting? What have you been attracting? If your answers are not to your liking, know that your conditions can change as quickly as your thoughts change. Radiate deliberately in order to attract the good things you desire because whatever you focus on, you will attract.

Your rich mindpower and radiations will go ahead of you and produce right opportunities, events and circumstances for wealth and success.

While you must think and act right, I believe that riches, wealth, and abundance are the result of 98% inner preparation (how you're thinking) and 2% outer action (what you're doing). If that belief really is true, and I believe it is, isn't it worth it to do some daily thinking on purpose in order to create the results you want on purpose?

Riches, Wealth & Abundance Exercise #1

Become aware of all of your thoughts and make note of the disempowering thoughts and feelings that are limiting you.

Do you say to yourself any of the following on a regular basis?

- "I can't afford it."

- "It's too much money."

- "I don't have enough."

- "There's never enough."

- "Everything is so expensive?"

Eliminate these negative thoughts and words. You may think your affirmations, what you say when you talk to yourself, are all positive, but beware that whatever you repeat to yourself over and over again is an affirmation, regardless of whether it is positive or negative. Be very cognizant of the words you are using. Replace them with "wealth decrees," intentional positive statements that say what you truly desire, and that serve you. Do them for just five minutes per day, and be sure to do them out loud. You can do them in the shower, while you're putting on makeup, or alone in the car. Here are a few of my favorites:

Wealth Decrees

- Everything and everybody prospers me now. I prosper everything and everybody now.

- I love the highest and best in all people! I now draw to myself the highest and best people (customers, clients, patients, etc.).

- Divine order is now established and maintained. Harmony reigns supreme!

- With praise and thanksgiving, I set the riches of God before me this day to guide, govern, protect, and prosper me. All things needful are now provided. My rich good becomes visible this day!

- My words are charged with prospering power.

- I give thanks that my financial income now increases mightily through the direct action of God's rich good.

- I give thanks for the immediate, complete payment of all financial obligations, now quickly and in peace.

- God's wealth is circulating in my life. His wealth flows to me in avalanches of abundance. All of my needs, goals and desires are met instantaneously for I am one with God and God is everything.

The Vacuum Law of Wealth

When I worked with the single moms, we worked with several prosperity laws, and this by far was a favorite. Nature abhors a vacuum, meaning that any space that's empty will soon be filled up. This principle is particularly true in the realm of wealth. If you want greater good, greater wealth, start forming a vacuum to receive it. The way to form your vacuum is to get rid of what you do not want, in order to make room for what you do want. If you have clothes, furniture, or objects in your home or office that no longer seem right for you, or even friends or acquaintances that are no longer empowering, begin moving these tangibles and intangibles out of your life. You are then creating a space for new and improved people and blessings to enter your life.

It is often difficult to know what you want until you get rid of what you do not want. If there is an experience, money or item you desire, and it has not appeared, it is possibly because you need to release and let go of something to make room for it.

Picture your current living environment as empty because you desire to move into a new one. Picture your current car clean and selling quickly and easily, as you desire to drive a new one. Many experts in success, including Napoleon Hill, Maxwell Maltz, and John Assaraf all tout the power of visualization. There is simply nothing easier than closing your eyes and envisioning how you'd like to live your life.

Whenever you dare to form a vacuum, something better then rushes in to fill that empty space.

Another vacuum you can form is with forgiveness, by forgiving others of their unkind deeds against you also creates a vacuum. You are letting go of negative feelings and in their place can come, if you let them, better and happier thoughts and feelings. Better yet, decide to let those negative thoughts and feelings go, and in their place, intentionally put some new and positive ones.

When a challenge is stubborn and doesn't seem to resolve itself over time, even with action on your part, it could be because there is a need for forgiveness. Ask yourself, whom do I need to forgive? If even only one person in a situation starts the action of forgiveness, all concerned will respond, and be blessed. It is then that a solution will come.

Release is Magnetic.

Start the flow of substance by graciously releasing, letting go, and blessing what you've released, including people, situations and things. Picture what you wish to create, and almost right away a magnetic influence will go to work for you.

Another way to invoke the vacuum law of wealth is by using your present visible substance by not withholding it. Releasing it by spending it freely will allow new channels of wealth to come to you.

Establishing and maintaining a prosperous attitude just as though your bounty were already completely visible is important at this point. This is not the time to talk lack, to withhold, or to practice stringent frugality. This is the time to use up the last of your financial assets, to the last penny, if necessary. If you withhold, talk about financial lack at this point, it can cost you double. Instead, "look up" mentally and give thanks for the substance you already have. Joyously declare, "This is the bounty of God and I send it forth with wisdom and joy."

Put your best foot forward. Wear your best clothes, look your best. Live as richly as possible on what you already have. Don't mention your current financial conditions, to anyone. Speaking of your lack of money and current limitation can keep you in financial lack and limitation. Never think of yourself as poor or needy. Do not ever talk about the fact that you're having a hard time or that you are short on cash. Just focus on the future, talk abundance, look your best, use your best china and silver, and eat by candlelight, even if you're eating macaroni and cheese!

As you form a vacuum, almost mysteriously, new channels of supply will appear to meet your needs. Money will come from out of nowhere, gifts will be given at just the right time, and you'll have everything you need just when you need it.

This process is not a one-time deal. You can and should continue to make room for your expanded good to come to you. There must be constant elimination of the old to keep pace with this growth. When you cling to the old, you hinder your advance or stop it altogether. Dare to form a vacuum now and invite the riches, wealth, abundance, and success you deserve!

Riches, Wealth & Abundance Exercise #2

Continue to create a vacuum by getting your home and office in order. Get rid of the things you do not want in order to make room for what you do want. Clean up the closets, the junk drawers, other drawers, the cabinets, and the shelves. Go through stacks of paper, boxes of documents and piles of magazines and recycle, throw out or shred anything you no longer need. Clutter isn't congruent with a clear path to abundance. I will say I always feel amazing after I've gotten everything in order and put a few trash bags outside the back door. It's so liberating and even when I've finished the task, I keep an eye out for anything else I can release because I find letting go and throwing things out so much fun.

The Creative Law of Wealth

Let's get down to the business of creating true wealth. Now that you've created a vacuum, you're ready to fill that vacuum with rich, new good through the creative law of wealth.

The Creative Law of Wealth contains three steps, which we've covered a bit already.

Step One: Create your life plan by writing out your desires concerning that plan, and by constantly expanding it.

Step Two: Mentally imaging that plan as fulfilled.

Step Three: Constantly affirming its perfect fulfillment.

There is nothing lukewarm or weak about true desire. It is intense and powerful. If properly developed and expressed, a strong desire always carries the power for success. The stronger your desire is for good, the greater the power of your desire to produce that good for you.

Release your deep-seated desires for riches, wealth, and abundance by centering your attention on one big goal at a time. Your big goal includes many smaller desires that are automatically fulfilled when the big one is achieved.

Write down your desires.

Make a list or draw up a plan, which you should feel free to change, revise, reform and rearrange as your ideas about it unfold. Writing out your desires and formulating a plan on paper clarifies the desires in your mind. The mind produces definite results only when it has been given definite ideas.

Get clear and specific about your desires: how you want to live better and how much more money you need.

Wealth is a planned result. It is the result of your deliberate thought and action. Without deliberate, consistent action, there will be no prosperous results on a consistent, permanent basis. Be as definite and specific as you can, so be sure to review, revise and update often.

If you are not clear about what it is you do want, begin to make lists about what you definitely don't want to do. On the bottom of that list write these words and declare out loud, "This too shall pass."

Write out your desires for the next six months, and then write out your desires for each of those six months. Each day, review your list to keep your mind focused on what you want. This exercise will make what's happening in your life right now much easier to deal with.

Then, each week, add or change your list, depending on the results you're getting and where you're being led to make changes. Spend at least 15 minutes a day pouring your verbal prayers (wealth decrees) upon your listed desires, and work daily on your list revising, changing, and expanding it.

Get very definite about the things you want to bring into your life. List the amount of money you wish to make for the day, week or month. List clothing you want to wear, trips you want to take, even the car you want to drive. Place a time limit and definite dates by which you wish the fulfillment of your desires. Do not wonder, doubt or question how it will come about, stay busy putting the creative laws of riches, wealth and abundance into action in these simple ways. You're looking for magic and miracles here, and humans don't create them. I believe we allow them.

These ideas may seem simple. Indeed, they are so simple the average person overlooks them in trying to find a more difficult way.

Make your list daily! At the end, write a note of thanks to God for the "divine fulfillment and the divine achievements." Review your list at the end of the day, include thank you notes to God for what was achieved.

Another note-writing technique that is helpful in getting bills paid: instead of resenting them as they arrive, write on the envelopes, "I give thanks for your immediate and complete payment. You are immediately and completely paid through the rich avenues of divine substance."

Riches, Wealth & Abundance Exercise #3

Make a list daily of what you wish to bring into your life in abundance. Work with it, and your wealth decrees every day.

The Imaging Law of Wealth

You've made your lists and are working with them daily. You've changed them, expanded them and revised them. Now there is another step you're ready to take. This is the time to invoke the imaging power of the mind. This law is almost magical and can work for you as, up to this point, it may have worked against you.

There has been quite a bit of study of the mind and how it works. It has been determined that anything a woman can imagine, she can create. The mental images we hold create our conditions and experiences. Our only true limitation comes from the negative use of imagination. If you have experienced, or are experiencing lack and limitation, it is because you first imagined lack and limitation. Here's the truth, if you're experiencing what you don't want to experience, it's because you've used your imagination to create those results instead of intentionally using your imagination to create the results you truly want. You've created those negative past experiences, but in the same way, on purpose, you can begin to dissolve those situations and experiences and create new ones!

Sometimes the imaging power of the mind produces immediate results for you. If the results take a bit longer, rest assured what is coming is bigger and better than you have imagined. The longer it takes your mental images to produce results, the bigger they will be.

Charles Fillmore once described the terrific power of the imagination when he wrote, "Imagination gives man the ability to project himself through time and space and rise above all limitations."

Your Master Plan is truly powerful, as you have written it on paper in the form of your six months, one month one week and daily goals. Now it is time to add imaging power to create success and wealth at a faster rate.

Your wealth map is a practical tool that you can make for any and all desired situations and experiences in life. The single moms from the first book loved making their wealth maps. These maps got their creative juices flowing to look through magazines and print out pictures from the Internet of the things they wanted to bring into their lives.

To create a wealth map, also known as a vision board, you'll need a poster board, glue-stick, and magazines with pictures of items, situations and conditions you want to create.

Be sure your images have the necessary details, so only use pictures and words that are clear and specific. Picture what you want exactly as you want it, and then dismiss the picture from your mind, knowing the results will manifest quickly and easily.

It is worth your time to spend time daily mentally

picturing what you want to create, staring at your wealth map, and expanding those pictures in your mind in as much detail as possible. Again, once your picture is clear, as it gradually will be you will need to take little or no action in order for results to come.

The law one of the most fascinating laws to work with!

The Wealth Law of Command

It is through the wealth law of command that you release the flood of good that has built up through your list-making and mental images.

The wealth law of command is your key to your dominion. The word command means "to have authority or control." As you speak definite words of wealth, you take control of your destiny and world with a feeling of authority and control that produces like results.

The secret of the law of command is this: a positive assertion of the good you wish to experience is often all that is needed to turn the tide of events to produce good for you swiftly and easily. When you dare to take control of a situation, it's amazing how quickly and easily results appear!

There is nothing new about using the law of command. In Genesis, the Lord used the law of command in creating the earth by commanding, "Let there be … and there was." (Genesis I)

Just like writing down your desires and using your mind to imagine them as true, the Law of Command is easy to use. Now that you've made lists of your desires and mentally imaged them through making a wealth map, it is time to release the substance of them into words of decree and command that move the ethers into action. Remember, what you say and see is what you get!

You make your world with words, so never underestimate the power of words. If you are not pleased with the world you have created with words of lack, limitation and hard times, you can immediately create a new world of limitless good and wealth for yourself by changing your words of command and decree.

The single moms I wrote about in *The Successful Single Mom* found the Law of Command one of the easiest and fastest to produce rich results for them. They took affirmative statements that met their needs and declared them over and over, out loud, for at least fifteen minutes per day.

Get a pack of brightly colored 3x5 cards and write out your affirmations, one on each card. Carry them in your purse or wallet. Say them out loud often through the day … I say them first thing in the morning, while I'm exercising, and in the shower. As I go throughout my day, I say them while driving. I say them to myself while waiting in line at the post office, bank, etc. I have one taped to my computer, checkbook, my bathroom mirror, the refrigerator, and underneath my speedometer in my car. Put them anywhere you are constantly focusing your attention, so you'll see them and be reminded to declare them often. Your subconscious mind will see them even when your conscious mind doesn't.

If you are in a relationship with a like minded person, you can use the power of affirmative command together. Together, you super-charge the prospering power of this law.

In your journal, you can write out your affirmations. Write a full page of one affirmation, as often as you can, daily if possible to impress on your mind what it is exactly you want to bring to pass immediately.

Watch all of your words. Doing wealth decrees every day does not overcome any and all of the negative self-talk you are using throughout the rest of the day. Just begin to become aware of what you're saying to yourself that isn't helping. Then stop saying negative things to yourself, and replace those thoughts and words with the deliberate and positive thoughts that will be helpful.

There are hundreds, if not thousands, of affirmative statements you can use that will command good to appear, and definite declarations should be used to meet definite needs.

For instance if your money supply is low, or if your purse or checkbook seems empty, in private declare aloud a number of times, "I bless you and bless you for the riches of God that are now being demonstrated in and through you."

Really important: it is good to begin the day with affirmative statements. They will help you gain control of your day. As you go throughout your day, dressing, driving, eating, or other activity, think thoughts of appreciation and blessing for all that you have and are experiencing.

Your decrees will produce satisfying results. I have not heard of one instance where a person conscientiously follows the method of daily affirmations and command for even a short time without producing satisfying results. Nor will a student of this work succeed if this law is omitted. You may find it embarrassing or beneath you to say wealth decrees, but I submit to you that financial challenge and indebtedness are far more embarrassing!

Your final step is release. Greater good has come to me, after long periods of inner work, when I felt guided to release it all of its perfect results. Happy changes in my personal and business circumstances, changes in location and more have all appeared after I worked inwardly, then turned loose, relaxed and let go.

CHAPTER TEN

ENJOY THE JOURNEY!

The whole journey into riches, wealth and abundance is so much more fun if you enjoy it. By now you've figured out that what I'm going to tell you is that before you can enjoy it, you must decide to enjoy it.

If you're behind on all of your bills, in a bad job, or not receiving support of any kind from your ex, it is understandable you would be less than enthusiastic about the future. There are lots of tools in this book for you to use to help turn that around. If you don't already have one, be sure to get a notebook or a journal or even use a Word document, to begin to create your future intentionally.

If not for yourself, do it for your kids!

You are the Model

I recently experienced something life-changing. My daughter's therapist asked to see me, and she created a visual rendering of my family which included an overview of my grandmother's relationship with my mother, and my mother's relationship with me.

It was eye opening to see that my mother had recreated in her relationship with me her own relationship with her mother. While I won't go into the details, it was not at all good. In fact, it was heartbreaking. The therapist explained that as children, we tend to model our parents. We truly do what we see. If we have loving parents who encourage our dreams and goals, who believe there's always an abundance of money, that's what we will then model for our children.

However, if you're like me, your parents didn't model those things, so what you're modeling may not be what you want to model. The good news is, and there's always good news, you get to change your now, your future, and your children's futures.

It all comes down to one important question:

Do you want your children to grow up and live the life you're living?

If not, the tools in this book can help you change what you're modeling, and that change will ultimately shape your children's destinies.

Break the Cycle

Whatever you saw modeled, like what I saw modeled, I'm sure there was some good in there. It's up to you to break any cycle of any part of your modeling that you don't want your kids to recreate as adults.

I do believe talking with a therapist is helpful. I've already expanded on my thoughts regarding having a coach. In addition to your friends and family who love you, it's always good to have that neutral person who will call you on your "stuff," help you see the truth about you (note: that you're amazing and capable), and get you to move forward in ways that are great for you and your kids.

I also believe making a mental shift about what's possible, making sure my feet match my lips, and taking steps in a positive direction every day is my responsibility, and now, it's yours, too.

Put Your Life, and Everything in it, into Perspective

I got "in trouble" with my editor for not using an editor with my previous books. Here's the thing: you don't know what you don't know. Hopefully, this book has opened your eyes to some possibilities about what you didn't know before. This leads us to, "when you know better, you do better."

Now that you have some knowledge and tools, you can take those, expand on them as you deem right for you, and take your life, riches, wealth, and abundance to new heights! What's truly important is that your life, from your perspective, is rich, that you love on your kids as much as you can every day, that you feel like you're raising them the best you can, that you're doing creative and fulfilling work that compensates you abundantly, that you're happy every day you wake up. Doing each of these is a rich life, in my humble opinion.

Progress not Perfection

What you can ensure you do is make progress. Taking steps in the right direction really is about making progress, not achieving perfection. I was so happy the day I realized that perfection was not possible, and that I could do something to the best of my ability, smile, and walk away happy. You can do the same. Do the best you can do, make as much progress as you can make, and be sure to laugh every single day. Being able to laugh at one's self is one of the greatest life gifts!

The best is yet to come!

And that is the absolute truth!

CHAPTER ELEVEN

YOUR KIDS CAN BE RICH, TOO!

The easiest and best way to ensure your kids will live a life of riches, wealth and abundance is to, as we've discussed, be an amazing model.

We all dream that our children will grow up to be independent, successful adults, able to support themselves, happy in their work, providing for their own families (and if necessary, us!).

Right alongside that dream is another dream: that our children are truly, deliriously happy.

Happy and rich – what's not to like?

These are terrific dreams, and I have those dreams for my own daughter.

It's difficult for our children to become rich, wealthy and abundant, but for reasons you may not think. The toughest part in that process is getting parents to believe in their children. Most kids are innately enthusiastic, confident and motivated, but their parents discourage them from acting on these innate feelings, especially about money.

Well-meaning moms (and dads) unconsciously act on their outdated and ambivalent beliefs about money, and it is these very beliefs that prevent their kids from prospering.

Parents who discourage their children from going for their dreams is astounding to me, and I believe that is because they're coming from a place of fear. It's important you put your fears in check and encourage your children to dream big dreams, and to go for their dreams.

If they want to be a musician, artist, actor or entrepreneur, encourage them! If they want to be a doctor, lawyer, or CPA, encourage that, too! If they want to open a vet clinic, antique store or car wash, help them to research the options, know the upsides and downsides and make an informed decision.

If you believe you're part of the 99% that's being kept down by the 1%, that's what you'll pass on to your children, but if you can embrace your children's unique talents and abilities, and teach them practical money and even business skills, you can become their best teacher. This education actually will bring you closer to your kids.

Our education system teaches our kids basic knowledge, but not some of the essential skills they need to know, such as how to manage time, create relationships, balance their checkbooks, capitalize on opportunities, and get organized (I could go on). All of those skills and abilities are essential for success.

While you're researching your new job or considering starting a new business, bring your kids in on the process as it's happening. Age-appropriate conversations get them to thinking, and having your kids encourage you is one of the greatest feelings ever.

If you're learning new financial skills, share with your kids what you're learning. When something happens as a matter of course in their home, kids accept what they see as reality and will adopt that as "what is" in their lives as they grow and mature.

My daughter assumes everyone's mom works from home, has her own business, and spends a lot of time on the phone. It's funny when she hears, "I'll call you on my break," or "I can't attend because I can't get off of work." I have had to explain to her that our home is not the norm.

Because of what she's witnessed her entire life, Lexi's already talking about how she's going to join me in my business. She constantly asks me questions and requests to learn more about what I do. She has already made several hundred dollars selling my books door-to-door in our neighborhood (you can read about that here: http://tinyurl. com/396ornq). Of course, she's only eleven so who knows what she'll grow up to do. What I do know is that she has an idea of what's possible, working for herself, and if she chooses to do so, she'll most likely be successful.

The thing is, as her mom, I'm not trying to control what she does. I'm giving her information and educating her on what her options are so she can make informed decisions when it's time for her to make her own decisions.

You can do the same with your kids, and trust me when I say that the rewards of this effort will surprise and amaze you, in a good way!

CONCLUSION

YOU ARE ON YOUR WAY TO WEALTH

You have my deepest gratitude for reading this book – thank you. I want to commend you for taking the time to read this book. In doing so, you have proved your commitment to yourself and your children. What comes next is going to be amazing for you. There will probably be a few moments of yucky thrown in for good measure, just to make sure you're paying attention and really committed to the amazing life you say you want.

What's next is truly up to you – and the possibilities are endless! From my heart to yours, I want you to hold out what for what you really want. Never settle or accept second best, go for what you want every single day.

You can do it, so do it. The best is yet to come.

To Your Success, Joy, and Happiness,

Honorée

RESOURCES

Blogs

Singlemommyhood.com: A thriving "neighborhood" where parents come daily for conversation and advice -- founded by two of the most popular single parent authors who know that single parenthood can be fulfilling, as well as incredibly demanding.

MsSingleMama.com: http://mssinglemama.com. Musings on life, love and motherhood.

Cassie Boorn: http://cassieboorn.com/. Super single mom writes about creating life on her terms.

Online Financial Resources

Mint.com

Bankrate.com

Yahoo! Finance: http://finance.yahoo.com.

WiseBread.com

Darci Poloni, Estate Planning Attorney:
http://www.polonilaw.com/about/.

Online General Resources

Mom Invented: Moms helping mom. http://www.mom-inventors.com/ Makes me want to invent something right away! The Mom Invented® brand has products that they manufacture and sell nationwide and, they offer education through Mom Inventor's Inc. Founder & CEO Tamara Monosoff's books. Her books teach entrepreneurs about how to launch and build their businesses. She also offers an intensive 4-week Power Mentoring Program offered approximately three times per year. The MomInvented. com community is free and offers both information and inspiration. You can find them on twitter: @mominventors and Facebook: http://www.facebook.com/mominvented.

Operation GI Jane. http://www.Operation-GIJane.org Operation G.I. Jane is a non-profit organization dedicated to supporting deployed single mothers in the U.S. military.

Single Mothers Online: http://www.singlemothers.org/.

The Successful Single Mom blog http://thesuccessfulsinglemom.blogspot.com/

Single Mom Reading Resources

You can find these books by click on their links, when available, or through Amazon(dot)com.

The Complete Single Mother: Best-selling self-help book

for single parents – ***The Complete Single Mother*** – now out in its third edition. Reassuring answers to your most challenging concerns.

Single Mom Seeking: A spunky tell-all about how to date and remain a dedicated parent, with lots of pitfalls and rewards — single-mom style. ***Single Mom Seeking*** was optioned in 2011 for a TV show.

The Single Moms Little Book of Wisdom: 42 Tidbits of Wisdom To Help You Survive, Succeed and Stay Strong by Cassandra Mack

My Single Mom Life: Stories and Practical Lessons for Your Journey by Angela Thomas

Helping Your Kids Cope with Divorce the Sandcastles Way by M. Gary Neuman & Patricia Romanowski

Business Opportunity Resources

Shaklee Corporation. On the web, visit http://honoree. myshaklee.com. For a real person I know personally, contact Galen Lahman at lahmans@embarqmail.com or 740-927-1191. Use reference ID: TA93601

You can find franchise information at: http://www.franchiseopportunities.com.

Additional Suggested Success Reading

Think & Grow Rich & Law of Success, by Napoleon Hill

Awaken the Giant Within by Anthony Robbins

<u>Success Principles</u> by Jack Canfield

<u>Go for No!</u> by Richard Fenton & Andrea Waltz

<u>The Secret</u> by Rhonda Byrne

Success Magazine

Any book by Norman Vincent Peale, Mark Victor Hansen, or John Maxwell.

Author's note: I'm not compensated in any way, with the exception of products you may purchase through Shaklee, by any of the above. It's just the good people, books and resources I've found in my research for <u>The Successful Single Mom</u> series.

NOT WITHOUT YOU

To my mastermind peeps ~ you know who you are. I remain in awe of you. Thank you for your love and support. I'm accomplishing more than I ever thought possible and I'm so grateful to you!

To the single moms ~ Thank you for your contribution to this book and to your fellow single moms. Women who work in concert and cooperation are the best!

To Lexi ~ Thank you for being such a wonderful daughter! You inspire me to be the best mom I can be. I love you with all of my heart.

To my wonderful husband ~ You were the person I was waiting for all this time. Thank you for being such an incredible blessing. Every great thing in my life, including this book, wouldn't exist without you. I love you.

To Greg Russell ~ Thank you for sharing your talents with my readers and me. You have a gift and I'm so glad we've connected!

Honorée

WHO IS HONORÉE

Honorée is a mega-successful leader of leaders; player-coach, entrepreneur, author, speaker, and mentor to professionals around the world, helping them grow their businesses and live amazing lives. She empowers others to dream big and go for what they truly want.

Author. Honorée is the author of The Successful Single Mom book series, Tall Order!, Master Strategies for Explosive Business Growth, including the upcoming The Successful Single Mom Gets Fit!

Personal Transformation Expert. She specializes in helping individuals and professionals achieve their maximum potential.

Turns Service Professionals into Rainmakers. Honorée gives seminars and conducts training programs on generating business, creating strategic partnerships and practicing exceptional business courtesy for service professionals. Her certified coaches teach her popular coaching class, The STMA (Short Term Massive Action) 100-Day Coaching Class for Professional Women and Young Professionals.

Inspires the Masses. Honorée is a source of inspiration, motivation and transformation through her books, radio shows, monthly informational tele-coaching, seminars, blogs, success interviews, television appearances, and online inspirational courses. She presents immediately applicable and practical procedures for focusing vision, goals and actions on the attainment of the life desired.

Former Successful Single Mom. Honorée is the proud mom of Lexi, a truly special 11-year-old sixth-grader who teaches her new things about success every day. She does her very best to live what she teaches … and she teaches it so she remembers to live it.

Still a Blissed Out Newlywed. Using the tools in this book prepared her to attract and marry her fantastic new husband, Byron Corder. Now married three years, so wakes up in awe and full of gratitude every day.

Single Mom Blog. Her blog empowers thousands of single moms,* providing tips, tools, strategies, ideas and recipes for making the most of yourself, your mommy-ness, and your life. Visit and subscribe at: http://thesuccessfulsinglemom.blogspot.com

*OK, not yet, but that's the vision. Since you've read this far, why don't you become a follower?

Honorée Enterprises, Inc.
Honoree@CoachHonoree.com
http://www.coachhonoree.com
Twitter: http://www.twitter.com/Honoree
Facebook: http://www.facebook.com/Honoree
Smashwords:
https://www.smashwords.com/profile/view/Honoree
My blog: http://Honoree.blogspot.com

#####